Chair Yoga For Seniors

Help Relieve Pain, Prevent Falls, and Boost Mobility for Greater Independence

Jackie Jacobs

Contents

Medical Disclaimer

This book goes through a number of different yoga poses. It is best to check with your doctor if you have any medical conditions or injuries to ensure certain poses are right for you.

Acknowledgments

To My Siblings

Who could've predicted that those feisty kids, battling over the last cookie or ever-elusive TV remote, would grow up to be best friends?

We've spent countless hours debating the critical issues of our time: Whose turn was it to wash dishes? Who misplaced the remote control (again)? And of course, which of us is truly Mom's favorite? (It's me, by the way.) Yet, the one thing that was never a debate was our unwavering support for each other.

Without you, this book would likely still be a mere thought, tucked away in the corner of my mind. Thank you for being you. I love you.

Introduction

In the last 10 years, how physically active would you say you were? As we get older, that part of our life tends to slow down, and ironically, the lack of physical activity will surely catch up to us at one point or another.

Believe it or not, the Centers for Disease Control and Prevention (CDC) (2023) states that seniors need at least 150 minutes of vigorous exercise per week. That's 30 minutes a day for 5 days. What's more, the CDC recommends that 2 days a week should be allotted to building muscle and that you should also include fitness routines designed to improve your balance. But why is this important for the older folks? Falling is a big concern among the senior population. Its results are not only costly to the individual if they suffer a severe injury, such as a broken leg, but it can also be fatal.

As we get older, our bodies feel it. Our joints ache more than they used to. If we suffer an injury, it takes longer to heal. You get the picture. A fitness routine can reduce your risk of falling and prevent injuries or, at the very least, reduce your recovery time. Thirty minutes a day may seem like a lot (or boring), but it's ultimately worth it for your health and wellness. This is why I love chair yoga; it's incredibly versatile! The number of poses is endless, which keeps your workout fresh and provides a different way to exercise without putting significant strain on the body. Plus, it helps improve balance and build muscle, which keeps us stronger for longer.

In most cases, people who have never done yoga automatically assume they must be flexible, perfectly balanced, and a graceful swan-like acrobat. However, despite the visualization, it's far from the truth. People who experience chronic pain or a chronic health condition are among the top groups to benefit significantly from yoga, specifically chair yoga. As yoga is a dynamic stretching routine, it can be a way to help you work through the pain or to improve your overall physical health that has become hindered by a chronic health condition.

Even so, if you don't have chronic pain or a chronic health condition, you may still find that your mobility is not quite what it used to be. For example, once upon a time, going up a flight of stairs probably took you less than a minute, and now it seems to take five minutes, going one step at a time. The problem with decreased mobility is that it makes getting around harder and may also reduce your motivation to get out and enjoy life. It may also increase your concerns about falling, especially if you have taken a tumble already.

In other cases, some turn to exercise because they want to lose or maintain weight. However, weight can be slightly more complex in our golden years, especially keeping it off. This could be from not being overly active over the years, or it could have been caused when mobility, chronic pain, or a chronic health condition came into your life. Whatever the reason is, it shouldn't be the reason it stops you from putting your health first.

That said, with our bodies slowing down and mobility issues making their appearance, we also find our energy levels have decreased. When energy levels drop, achieving goals and engaging in activities we once enjoyed can feel more challenging. Those activities could be a walk around the block with our spouse, or it was once going to play lawn bowling while socializing at the lawn bowling club on a nice summer day.

Your body changing may seem frustrating at times, but it's important to remember that it's a natural way of life, and you can find the spark to your energy or find a way to manage your pain through chair yoga.

Yoga is like a breath of fresh air. It brings your mindfulness back to the forefront, reenergizing you and getting you back to what is important. You don't need mobility to be something that stops you from those walks or fears that you will fall over and injure yourself. While yoga gives you a different way to move, it has many proven benefits to help your overall health and reach your goals, regardless of what those goals may be.

Chair yoga is great for seniors because it allows you to practice this ancient exercise form in a way your body can handle. It will enable you to remain active, even if you have issues with your mobility and flexibility. It also allows you to work through some poses if you have a limited range of motion. All in all, chair yoga helps you prevent strain and injuries.

As you do yoga from a chair, it may feel awkward and different compared to regular yoga on a mat on the floor, but remember that it prevents you from getting injured and should not dissuade you from trying the different poses. I will show you how to get the most out of your routines and safely from your chair as it supports you.

In this book, we'll also look into warmups and cooldowns that will serve your body well so you can easily and confidently move through the various yoga flows. When you take the time to warm up and cool down, you can prepare your body for the work to come in addition to giving it what it needs to recover. Yoga is gentle and nothing like lifting weights or jogging, but it is essential as it contributes to getting the most out of your routine.

Throughout this book, I will give you step-by-step instructions on performing various yoga flows that you can fit into your day in 10 minutes or less. The routines will present the following benefits:

- improve balance
- ease joint and arthritic pain
- increase mobility
- build strength
- improve flexibility
- boost your cardio through cardio exercise
- boost your metabolism to help with weight loss

I have been a yogi for a while now. Having been through some injuries myself, including a shoulder injury that led me to have surgery, I have found that yoga has helped me along the way to help me recover from that injury and others. Around the same time as my surgery and rehabilitation, I began to help my grandparents and my parents as they moved into their golden years. So my injury ignited a new purpose, and I am glad to be your person to guide you through your fitness journey.

I also love that yoga has brought mindfulness into my life. Unfortunately, in a world where life is busy and sometimes chaotic, it is easy to get lost in the shuffle between appointments and events. While these yoga flows are short workouts that can be implemented in 10 minutes (short enough for a quick break on a busy day), I hope that as you get used to the flow, you find a sense of empowerment to go through the movements longer as you need.

The more movement you can implement into your life, the more you can focus on what is important to you. Our bodies are inevitably going to change, and we are going to get older. Aging is a beautiful process that can be embraced with new clarity when we can reclaim some of our abilities. You don't need to think about running a marathon. Imagine how a walk around the block will feel when your body can handle the movement because you took the time to work on your mobility, flexibility, and range of motion through yoga. Maybe it's not a walk around the block but the ability to play with your grandchildren. Whatever is important to you, yoga can bring it back into your life and in a new light.

1
What is Chair Yoga?

According to the National Center for Complementary and Integrative Health (NCCIH), the popularity of yoga among seniors in America is growing, with "6.7 percent" of seniors aged 65 and up practicing yoga in 2017 "compared to 3.3 percent in 2012, 2.0 percent in 2007, and 1.3 percent in 2002" (NCCH Clinical Digest for Health Professionals, 2020).

There are many reasons why people begin to practice yoga. Some want the benefits of mindfulness as the practice heavily focuses on breathing. For others, they seek out yoga because they want to improve their overall flexibility. Within the aging population, however, yoga offers seniors an accessible way to exercise in a gentle form. That said, it can feel daunting for some who want to get into a yoga practice if getting up and down from the floor for various movements is a challenge. So, what is chair yoga exactly?

Chair yoga is a form of yoga practiced as you sit in a chair. As you would find in regular yoga performed on a mat, chair yoga has a sequence of poses strung together. You move your body in a specific way through each pose and hold the position before moving into the next yoga pose. Additionally, chair yoga involves movements that challenge your balance. While yoga, in general, is a gentle form of exercise, chair yoga is much milder and more accessible to those who require additional support and ways to adjust yoga poses based on the needs of the individual. Chair yoga is an excellent option for you if you

- have arthritis that impacts your range of motion.
- have difficulty balancing.
- have difficulty moving your body for any other reason.

Elements of Chair Yoga

Chair yoga and regular yoga share similar elements, including

- warmup poses.
- standing poses performed with the support of a chair.
- yoga poses focused on the lower body.
- a relaxing posture to cool you down from your yoga practice.

How to Do Chair Yoga

Yoga's mindful practice allows you to focus on your body and how it feels through the movement of the varying poses while breathing deeply. Your focus on your body will tell you how a pose feels, whether comfortable, uncomfortable, or causing pain. By keeping your movements focused and gentle, you'll be able to increase the intensity over time by building your strength and confidence.

Once you get the hang of a flow, yoga is like dancing. Try not to be rigid in the movements as you move from one yoga pose to another. While moving your body through the postures, ensure you deeply inhale and exhale, as breathing will encourage your joints to relax. Doing so will bring your mind to focus on how you feel through the posture and will allow you to connect to the more profound benefits of the pose.

As you move through the poses on your chair, keep your spine tall to avoid slouching. Other things to remember with maintaining your posture are to ensure your knees are stacked over your ankle, your feet remain flat on the floor, and avoid bouncing or jerking your feet.

If you have osteoporosis or osteopenia, it's best to avoid twisting movements or forward bends as bones are weakened due to these conditions and are more susceptible to fractures. If you do lean forward in a pose, ensure you bend from your hips instead of your waist and maintain a straight spine.

The Benefits of Chair Yoga

Any form of an active lifestyle has many benefits, hence why exercise is the best medicine. But, I recognize that not everyone can move in the same way they used to, which may lead them away from remaining physically active. What I love about chair yoga, and I've said this before, is how accessible it is. Regardless of your limitations, chair yoga can help you regain your strength and much more!

Better Flexibility

Think about a time when you went to perform a task, such as picking up the paper, and you felt a sudden twinge or spasm. Did the pain cause you extreme discomfort for the next couple of days? If it did, you're not alone. One of the earlier things we lose is our flexibility. It's ironic when you think about it because we use flexibility in nearly everything we do. But as our bodies age, they become more rigid and stiff. Contrarily, the loss of flexibility is not because we are aging (though it is easy to assume that's the reason); we lose our flexibility because we stopped using it to its full capability.

That said, stretching, bending, twisting, and moving easily is vital in all life aspects. Flexibility allows us to pick up that newspaper or enjoy any other activity without the repercussion of moving a specific way. So while you may feel like your flexibility is lost and you'll never get it back, that thought is untrue. As your body becomes challenged through chair yoga, you can regain flexibility and improve your range of motion and mobility.

Improved Strength

Yoga is considered a dynamic stretching routine, but don't be fooled. Your muscles need to work to hold the poses, thus building strength through your yoga practices. Improved strength will help you balance better, minimizing the risk of falling. Better strength also helps prevent injuries to support your bones and joints. Overall, having strength is essential as it makes your daily activities easier and doable.

Improved Bone Health

Bones are more than just our foundational skeleton. Bones are living tissues that go through a process known as remodeling. Every 10 years, our bones will regenerate to remove old bone to make room for new bone tissue. This process helps to keep the bones and their cells strong and healthy so that we can get more calcium supply throughout our body.

However, as we age, our bones' regeneration cycle slows down. It could be due to genetics, exercise, nutrition, or hormonal loss. Unfortunately, we can't change our genes (as much as we would love to), but we can control what we do to improve our overall health through nutrition and exercise.

Although some yoga poses are dynamic, others, such as Warrior II, are isometric contractions where we remain in a posture for a moment or two. This means that the muscles helping to hold the pose don't change.

Exercises that support load-bearing movements to build stronger muscles can also help to slow down bone loss. Likewise, yoga asanas challenge your body to hold the pose as you put weight on your bones. While learning how to do yoga from your chair, you'd be surprised how you can put weight on your bones to help strengthen them (along with your muscles).

Better Balance

Balance is crucial, from stepping onto a curb to bending down to pick something off the floor. Yoga helps with movement, coordination, balance, and focus because you learn to find balance through movement instead of focusing on being still in the yoga poses. As you improve on transitioning from one pose to the next, you'll be able to maintain your overall balance.

When considering maintaining your balance, even from a chair, you want to consider these three factors: alignment, strength, and attention.

For alignment, you want to ensure your center of gravity is aligned with your body so that you can physically balance. In addition, being aligned with your center of gravity means you have an improved self-awareness, especially concerning proprioception, when you are fully aware of your body in its space, strengthening your ability to coordinate.

As yoga works to improve your overall strength and attention, these, combined with balance, allow you to find, hold, and adjust your alignment as needed. It also means that if something may be causing you to feel a little topsy-turvy, you can modify the pose as needed so you don't tumble off your chair.

Improved Posture

While you may be part of an older generation that isn't always relying on technology, we still seem to be spending more time hunched over than we used to be. Since yoga can improve your flexibility and mobility, it shouldn't surprise you that yoga can also enhance your posture. The benefits from this can release commonly tight muscles, such as the hamstrings, while improving the mobility of your spine.

Pain Management

Exercise is excellent for pain management as working out encourages your body to release endorphins. Through chair yoga, your focused breathing through the poses and the gentle movement can help you work through the pain as you work to regain the range of motion and stretch your muscles.

Arthritis

Arthritis is problematic for many seniors. Not only does it cause pain and stiffness, but it can also impair your range of motion, cause swelling, and in some cases, redness. Through yoga practices, you can reduce the pain associated with arthritis which will reduce joint pain and improve your joints' flexibility and functionality.

Lower Back Pain

Did you know that Americans spend about $50 billion on seeing doctors regarding lower back pain (Contie, 2011)? That's a lot of money to spend trying to figure out what is happening with someone's back! However, interestingly, Dr. Karen J. Sherman, who led a team of researchers from the Group Health Research Institute in Seattle, ran a clinical trial with 228 adults, all of whom had been dealing with moderate lower back pain for three months.

The groups were split into three groups. Two groups were assigned to do 75-minute yoga classes or stretching exercises with a physical therapist over 12 weeks. The remaining group was given a self-care book outlining back pain and suggested an exercise routine and lifestyle changes to help reduce and manage their lower back pain.

After three months, the two groups participating in the yoga and stretching found their lower back pain significantly improved compared to those who received the self-care book. In addition, some of those in the yoga and stretching groups found they were not taking medication to manage their pain as often. Dr. Sherman told Contie (2011) that "yoga and stretching can be good, safe options for people willing to try physical activity to relieve their moderate low back pain."

Weight Control

Yoga may not be considered a traditional form of aerobic exercise, but certain types of yoga can be more physical than others, such as Vinyasa Yoga.

Vinyasa Yoga connects each pose using breathing techniques, which means you are constantly moving, which helps you to burn more calories. It is typically offered at hot yoga studios, but you can do this type of yoga from a chair too.

If one of your goals on your yoga journey is to lose weight, try incorporating a more active type of yoga practice at least three times a week and balance it with more gentle flows on other days.

Mental Health and Well-Being

Any form of exercise can boost your mood because it reduces your stress hormones and, as mentioned earlier, releases the endorphins that make you feel great. Throughout yoga practices, there is a heavy emphasis on breathing. Taking deep breaths can calm your nervous system, help relieve stress, and leave you feeling like you have more control over your life. That's not to say that yoga is a cure-all for mental health, but allowing yourself to be present and mindful can go a long way to having you feel mentally better.

Better Energy

As a lack of energy is a common complaint among seniors, consistent yoga practice can help to boost your mental and physical energy. I love that yoga gives me mental clarity, especially if I do my yoga practice first thing in the morning. It also helps me feel more alert since some mornings can be hard to function, especially during the long winter months! If that sounds like you, consider implementing your yoga practices in the morning so you can kickstart your day the right way!

Boost Cardiovascular Health and Functioning

Cardio or lifting weights doesn't need to be the only form of exercise to boost your heart rate to improve your cardiovascular health. Yoga can do the same for you without the added stress you might get from jogging, walking briskly, or lifting heavy weights.

As regular yoga practice enhances your overall mental health and reduces stress, it can also reduce inflammation caused by the stress hormone cortisol to improve your heart health. In addition, reducing stress and maintaining weight or boosting weight loss can also help lower blood pressure, minimizing the risk of heart disease.

Improved Immune System

Stress does a lot to our bodies. It can cause inflammation, impact our nervous system, and much more. When we are highly stressed, we open the door for illnesses and viruses to come in and knock us down for a few days. As we all know, being sick is no fun!

Though research is still developing to see how yoga can improve our immune system, researchers like Falkenberg et al. (2018) have seen a direct connection between long-term regular yoga practice and improving the immune system's functionality. It also comes down to how yoga can fight inflammation caused by stress to enhance cell-mediated immunity.

Improved Sleep

Ah, there is nothing more than waking up from a restful sleep. However, unfortunately, as we get older, our sleep patterns seem to get more interrupted. It could be due to several factors, such as

- restless leg syndrome
- medications
- sleep apnea
- changes to the circadian rhythm
- chronic pain
- insomnia
- overall poor sleeping habits

Regular physical activity can help you fall asleep and stay asleep. However, the aftereffects of working out, plus the mindfulness provided by yoga, can help you improve your sleeping patterns. Sleeping well can give you a more positive outlook and motivate you to get things done during the day.

A Former Non-Yogi Turned Yogi

When I first spoke to my friend Jane about writing a book on chair yoga, she told me that yoga was something she had yet to be interested in for the longest time. Like many others, she had preconceived notions that she wasn't flexible enough to handle yoga, let alone her mind is a busy body, and trying to quiet it down during a yoga session was a challenge for her.

However, my enthusiasm for yoga sparked her interest in learning more about it.

At the same time we chatted, Jane mentioned that she had been looking for other ways to work through her injuries; she decided to try yoga again, following a yoga video through her fitness streaming provider. After the first session, she had an ah-ha moment. She realized there was no need to be perfect while doing yoga, and she could laugh when she nearly fell over thanks to the speed wobbles.

Since that first yoga session, Jane has incorporated yoga into her fitness routine at least twice weekly to maintain her flexibility and mobility through other activities, such as running.

In addition, Jane has found that yoga has brought a new level of being mindful into her world. She finds that her busy brain finds time to calm down for at least 30 minutes so she can focus on her body, the movement of the poses, and the savasana portion of her practice. It's been a big game changer for Jane and her physical and mental health.

Chair yoga is great for seniors, but it's even better when you know how to get the most out of your yoga routines. In the next chapter, you will discover how to get into the right mindset before practicing yoga and how you can get the most out of your yoga routines physically.

2

How to Get the Most Out of Your Yoga Routine

 Yoga is the ultimate practice. It simultaneously stimulates our inner light and quiets our overactive minds. It is both energy and rest. Yin and Yang. We feel the burn and find our bliss. –BODi SuperTrainer Elise Joan

How to Get Into a Good Mindset Before Yoga

Let's consider this truth: Without understanding the intentions underlying your goal in chair yoga practices and how you plan to accomplish it, your yoga routine might lack effectiveness and motivation. To put it simply, Merriam-Webster (n.d.) explains that a 'goal' represents the desired outcome of your efforts, while 'intention' refers to the planned actions toward reaching that goal.

Your goal could be anything from increased flexibility to better mobility or perhaps a more relaxed state of being attained through your yoga practice. Recognizing your 'endgame' is crucial, yet, without the accompanying intention, there's a risk your goals may fall short or remain unfulfilled. It's essential not just to work towards your goal, but also to understand and embrace the intention that fuels it. This intention serves as the deep-seated connection between your mind and body and your desired outcome.

When setting an intention, you are clearly stating what you hope to achieve through your actions. It's your personal commitment to shaping your journey. It allows your mind to concentrate on the present, helping you comprehend who you are, what you're doing, and why you're doing it. Intentions act as a guiding beacon, keeping you aligned with the larger picture.

As you achieve your goals, guided by your intentions, you'll experience a surge of self-satisfaction. Moreover, you'll prove to yourself that you're capable of accomplishing what you set your mind to, which in turn bolsters your mental well-being.

What does this mean for getting into a good mindset regarding yoga? If you have ever attended a yoga class, you may have heard the instructor invite you to set an intention for your practice. Maybe it is something you've done where you decide what your purpose or hope is throughout the practice.

There is an important reason why instructors ask us to set an intention. They are essential to all mindful practices, including yoga and meditation. Your set intention for your practice does not need to be a long phrase (though if you choose to use a phrase, you're welcome to), but one word can align with your physical and mental energy.

Purposeful Intention-Setting

Before we talk about purposeful intention setting, I want to point out that setting an intention is not exclusive to meditation and yoga practices. They can be lifelong intentions or short-term (such as the next day or next hour).

Toli et al. (2015) found that our goals are often achieved when intentions are set alongside the goal. They influence our steps to get where we want to be in various parts of our lives. For example, you may set a goal for yourself to walk 30 minutes each day to improve your cardiovascular health. Ensure your intentions are specific and actionable, or the goal will be lost. However, for your yoga sessions, your intentions should help you focus on what you can control, such as your energy and keeping your mind in the present. Here are some other examples of intentions you could set for yourself in your yoga practice:

- be kind to yourself
- give yourself grace
- be present and refocus wandering thoughts
- use gentle movements to ease pain
- avoid comparing yourself to others

Declare Your Intentions

Whether internally or on a piece of paper, declare your intentions. Having it out there in the universe feels empowering and holds you accountable for what you want to do.

Be Clear

Whatever you want to achieve, be clear about what it is. Clarity makes it easier to focus your energy on where it needs to be.

Ensure Your Intentions Are Positive

As mentioned earlier, you can set your intentions for anything. It doesn't need to be solely focused on yoga. But, whatever intention you set for yourself, make it a positive one. For example, I will be patient with my body today.

Don't Complicate Your Intentions

The intentions you set for yourself and your yoga practice do not need to be attached to lofty goals. They should be something that you can realistically act upon. For intention setting and your yoga practice, you could set an intention for yourself to be fully present and connected to the poses you will do today.

Overcoming Self-Doubt

Self-doubt may want to try and creep in, but questioning whether you are doing it correctly is normal. Interestingly enough, when we set an intention for ourselves, our ego might want to chime in and say, "Oh yeah? Are you sure about that?" The ego can be our own worst critic from time to time, especially when it is casting its judgments. However, the ego is also how we can better understand ourselves and the experiences that come with it.

When your ego wants to chastise you, it can be hard to shake the limiting beliefs accompanying negative thoughts. When you cannot shake them off, it can impact how well you can execute your yoga session (or anything else), leading to even more inner criticism. If it sounds like a vicious cycle, it's because it is. If we allow internal judgments to tell us we can't do something, you'd be surprised at how easily we can find reasons why we can't. For example, if mobility in your shoulders is a significant issue for you and makes it difficult to lift your arms over your head, you'll believe that you can't do yoga because of that factor (and your brain may also tell you more reasons why).

Regardless of self-doubt, remembering why you set an intention in the first place and keeping it at the forefront of your mind can keep you on the right track. In yoga, there is no right or wrong. It isn't about being an acrobat doing wild balancing poses or being the most flexible yoga student. Instead, the focus should be connecting your mind and body to their overall best health and calming your mind.

Before you start any yoga session, focus on why you want to practice yoga today, whether it is to manage your pain, improve your range of motion, or something else—knowing why will help you work toward a bigger goal and keep you in alignment with your intention.

Tips to Set Your Yoga Intentions

Anyone can go into any form of exercise with a goal in mind. For example, some people exercise because they feel like couch potatoes and want to get back in shape. That sounds pretty straightforward, and keeping it isn't a challenging goal as long as you have the right exercise mindset. It's no different for chair yoga. Here are some simple steps to keep your perspective in the right place so you will keep up with your chair yoga routine.

Set Practical Expectations

What do you want to get out of your yoga sessions? That's the first question you should ask yourself, as it will help you figure out your goals for your yoga routine. If you're new to yoga, don't stress about perfecting all the moves or flowing smoothly between them. Instead, focus on a simple physical goal and try to understand why you've set this goal for yourself. Once you're clear about what you're trying to do, you'll find it easier to achieve, and then you can try something more challenging. It's like climbing a ladder. Each rung is a goal you're aiming for, and the steps you take to climb up are your strategy to reach it.

Sticking to your yoga routine can be tough, especially on days when you're not feeling your best. Maybe you didn't sleep well, or your body's sore, and moving is tougher than usual. On those days, it's easy to think, *ah, I'll just skip it. It won't matter if I miss one day.* But it does matter. When you let yourself off the hook for a day, you're telling yourself your goal isn't important, even when doing yoga is one of your favorite ways to stay fit.

Avoid the Pressure

Not every yoga session is going to go flawlessly. You could have done the same yoga routine hundreds of times, and then there is that one day when you can't seem to manage any of the asanas.

Putting pressure on yourself to execute the movements flawlessly, even from the first go around, can set you up for failure.

Likewise, if it's one flow you've done several times, and today it's just not going the way you want, let it go. Be kind, patient, and compassionate with yourself, and be okay if you have some limitations that may be holding you back for today's yoga practice. Instead of being frustrated with your current limitations, focus on how to work through them so they are not obstacles. Don't let anything discourage you just because it didn't go how you wanted it to today.

Have Fun

This is the most critical good mindset tip! Have fun! So what if you have speed wobbles because your chair is a little unstable, or you missed a part of the sequence? It happens! Smile or giggle it off and keep going!

Making Your Yoga Routine Work for You

Now that we know that setting intentions is how you will get yourself into the right mindset for your yoga practice. Having a good mindset and understanding your intentions to reach your goals will allow you to get the most out of your yoga routine and make it work for you and your needs.

Let Your Breath Be Your Dancing Partner

One of the first things you must establish while practicing yoga is to let your breath lead you. Many people think that yoga is all about the poses, but the breath is the partner to the movement to achieve each asana. The breath is like a dance partner so to speak. So let your breath lead you into the movement as the gentleman does in ballroom dancing.

See the Lessons in Metaphors

As your body and breath dance together to get to each pose, imagine each asana as a metaphor for your life. For example, in a tree pose (even from a seated position), visualize the difficult aspects of your life and how learning to master the pose can give your strength and courage beyond the chair. When you can see the lessons through the metaphors, you'd be surprised how positively your outlook on life can change!

Explore Basic Poses

As you begin to master some of the basic asanas, it can feel easy to shift your focus to improving more complex yoga poses that can test your flexibility and physical strength. However, focusing more on the difficult asanas can create a disconnect between the breath and the mind and body when we don't practice a pose we know well in a new way.

As you learn to see poses as metaphors, let them lead you to a new way to explore and reconnect to a basic yoga pose with something new. It will allow you to see the fine details and redefine the bigger picture you are trying to create from your practice.

Honor Yourself and Listen to Your Body

Your yoga practices will evolve consistently, so listening to yourself is essential. For example, some days, you may need a yoga practice that provides more restorative benefits, while others may need something more energetic. All you need to remember is to be honest with yourself and listen to the inner voice to honor what you need from your practices.

Your body will tell you what it needs when you listen to it. It will also tell you when something feels uncomfortable or is causing pain. If you are more concerned about how the pose looks and try to work through the pain, you could wind up with an injury, defeating why you practiced yoga today. As part of honoring yourself, it also means to take care of yourself. Find self-awareness to detect when a pose does not feel great, such as holding your breath. It will tell you to find a neutral position to allow your body a moment to reset.

Practice Yoga in a Distraction-Free Zone

A big part of all yoga practices is being present, entirely focused, and not allowing your inner chatter to squabble so loudly that you're not focused on the yoga movements. Before you start your yoga practice, clear all distractions preventing you from getting the most out of your practice. That means going to the bathroom before you begin, wearing comfortable clothes that allow you to move easily, keeping your pets out of your space, and keeping your hair out of your face.

Speaking of other distractions, put your cell phone aside (if you have one) and anything else that could connect you to the outside world. All of that can wait. The time you set aside to practice yoga needs to be respected, and when you have a phone pinging for your attention, it will make you lose focus on what is essential in your session.

Practice Gratitude

Be grateful for getting yourself onto your chair or mat and into the present. Feeling gratitude will enhance your yoga practice and follow you beyond your session.

Relaxation Techniques

In this interactive element, we will explore several techniques to help you set your mindset for yoga. Different relaxation techniques are an excellent way to help you manage stress levels—so they aren't just about doing things you enjoy or having peace of mind. They're also helpful for your yoga practice so that you can bring the true meaning of mindfulness onto your chair or mat.

Practicing relaxation techniques have a variety of benefits, including:

- lowering blood pressure
- slowing heart rate
- bringing your breathing to an average pace
- improving digestion
- managing blood sugar levels
- reducing stress hormones
- increasing blood flow to your muscles
- decreasing chronic pain and muscle tension
- improving sleep quality
- improving mood
- improving focus
- boosting confidence to handle whatever lemon is thrown at you

Breath Focus

Breath focus is one of the best relaxation techniques you can try. In this technique, you will focus on taking long, slow, deep breaths.

1. Find a comfortable position to sit in your chair.
2. Rest one hand on your heart and the other on your belly.
3. Take a long inhale, feeling the air fill your lungs and belly.
4. Exhale slowly through your nose or let it out through your mouth and repeat for five minutes, remaining present for each breath.

Body Scan

A body scan is a relaxation technique done alongside breath focus and works to relax your muscles. This relaxation technique helps enhance your awareness of the mind-body connection. By taking a few minutes of deep breathing, you can focus on one area of your body or several muscles to mentally release the tension you may be holding.

To do a body scan, tense your muscles from your toes up to your neck and head, holding for five seconds before releasing for 30 seconds. This method will allow you to feel where you have the most tension so that you can focus on letting it go.

Visualization

In visualization as a relaxing technique, you will form mental images that will take you on a visual journey to a place that brings your mind to a calm and peaceful state.

To use visualization as a relaxing technique, try to use as many senses as possible. For example, if you imagine yourself at your cabin in the woods, visualize the sound of the breeze moving through the trees and the sound of the water lapping against the dock. Whatever scene brings you peace, use that to boost the relaxed feeling.

Performing warmup and cooldown exercises is another way to get the most out of your yoga routine and stay safe and prevent injury during exercise. In the next chapter, you will discover how to warm up and cool down before and after your chair yoga routine.

3
Warmup and Cooldown Exercises

To warmup and cooldown or to not? Warming up and cooling down seems to be a big question among many people, and whether it is a critical element of any workout, whether it be jogging, playing a sport, or yoga and chair yoga.

Johnny Lee, M.D., who is the director of the Asian Heart Initiative at the New York City Langone Medical Center and president of the New York Heart Associates in New York City, says that "warming up before any workout or sport is critical for preventing injury and prepping your body" (American Heart Association editorial staff, 2014). So how does a warmup prepare your body? Taking 5 to 10 minutes to warmup will help to dilate your blood vessels so that your muscles have oxygen. It also helps to increase your body temperature to enhance flexibility and efficiency. In addition, by warming up, your body can gradually increase your heart rate instead of going from your resting heart rate to an intense one in seconds, minimizing the stress that would otherwise be put on your heart.

Likewise, when you cooldown, you allow your heart rate to return to normal so that the blood flow and oxygen do not suddenly become cut off once your workout is complete. When you don't take the time to cooldown, you risk getting cramped muscles and feeling dizzy. So even though yoga is a gentle workout, you should also spend at least five minutes cooling down so your body recognizes the exercise is ending.

Warming Up for Chair Yoga

With us focusing on chair yoga, you may think you don't need to warmup because it's not like you will be running off to the races. But, by warming up for chair yoga, you are preparing your muscles for the yoga poses to come later in your yoga practice. The warmup is an opportunity to slowly ease your muscles into the movements, preventing the risk of injury and boosting your overall practice. It should only take no more than 10 minutes so that your blood can flow to your muscles.

Think of your warmup for your yoga practice as a moving meditation. Too often, we move about in our day without much thought—like a hamster on its wheel. It's tradition for most yoga practices to begin with sun salutations to greet the sun and move our body with breathing techniques to put our mindset in a good place. Doing so will allow us to move freely and efficiently because we have taken the time to link our bodies to the movement. It will also bring clarity to our minds and a more positive outlook.

While warming up for your chair yoga session, move through the flow slowly and gradually as your body feels warmer. Your pace may change each time you cycle through the exercise. Listen to your body and breath to ensure you connect the two as you move your body through each yoga warmup. Let's take a look at some warmup movements you can do before you start your chair yoga session. Before you begin, ensure you have a sturdy chair with a back that is not on wheels.

Mountain Pose

One of the most commonly used poses is the Mountain Pose, and while it is a neutral seated position, it has various benefits! It's a foundational pose used in yoga to start a pose or routine. It helps improve your muscle imbalances and posture and boosts your awareness to see what other areas in your body may be holding tension. It's a simple pose to learn:

1. Sit in your chair with your feet hip apart and your hands resting on your thighs or knees.
2. Inhale to engage your core and lift your spine.
3. As you exhale, imagine your body is rooting itself to the ground, feeling your sit bones pushing into the chair's seat. Engage your legs as you press firmly into all four corners of your feet.
4. Pull your shoulders down and back as you take another deep inhale.

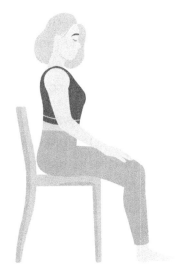

Mountain Pose

5. Hold for one minute.

Mountain Pose with Arms Up

This seated mountain pose has a new challenge as you lift your arms above your head. It's a great move to relax your shoulders and upper back while stabilizing your shoulder joint.

1. Sit in your chair with your legs hip-distance apart and your hands resting on your thighs or hanging by your side.
2. Inhale and bring your arms up overhead. Lace your fingers together as you keep your index fingers and thumbs out so you point directly to the ceiling.
3. Exhale and roll your shoulders away from your ears. Stay with your arms clasped above your head for five breaths.
4. Release and gently let your arms return to your sides.

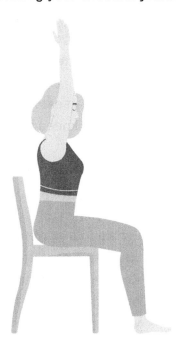

Mountain Pose With Arms Up

Sun Salutation

As we learned earlier, sun salutations are traditionally used at the start of a yoga practice. It may be a precursor to an excellent yoga practice, but it's truly a beautiful characteristic of a yoga practice with many great benefits.

Sun salutation, also known as *Surya Namaskar* in Sanskrit, means you are taking the time to bow down and show gratitude to the sun. It is a way for us to disconnect from the busyness of our lives and be present in our practice. I also want to show gratitude toward the sun for blessing us with another day of life around the sun.

As for a warmup, the sun salutation is an opportunity to open up all areas of your body to leave you feeling more balanced for your yoga practice. Here's how to do it:

1. Begin in a seated mountain pose (a neutral position) with your knees stacked over your ankles, hip-distance apart.
2. As you inhale deeply, lift your arms over your head, stretching them upwards like you are trying to touch the sky.
3. Exhale in a prayer pose as you bring your hands to your heart center.
4. Keeping your hands in the same position, fold forward by hinging at your hips and rounding your spine. Open your hands to reach toward the floor, resting your hands on your shins, ankles, or floor.
5. Inhale and roll up, imagining your vertebrae stacking on one another with your head lifting last.
6. Roll your shoulders so they are pulled away from your ears.

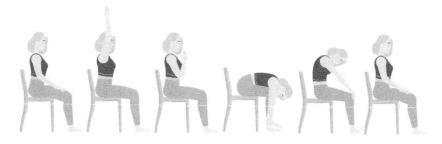

Seated Sun Salutation

Seated Cat-Cow

The cat-cow stretch is a movement that involves moving your spine from a rounded position to an arched one in conjunction with a breathing technique. By flexing and extending the spine through this movement, you allow the circulation around your discs to be improved, releasing any tension or pain in your lower back and spine and improving your posture. The cat-cow movement also helps to stretch your hips, abdomen, and chest muscles. Here's how to do it:

1. Begin in a seated mountain pose with your knees stacked over your ankles, hip-distance apart. Place your hands on your knees.
2. As you inhale deeply, arch your back to create this yoga pose's "cow" position. If it is comfortable enough, you are encouraged to deepen the arch of your back by extending your neck to look at the ceiling.
3. As you exhale, begin to round your back for "cat," pulling your belly button toward your spine and looking down at your belly.

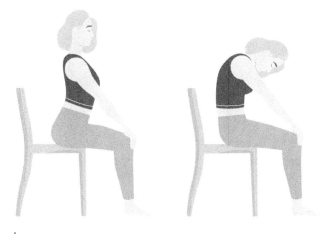

| Seated Cat-Cow Pose

Forward Bend

Whether from a chair or standing, forward bends are an excellent way to stretch and lengthen your hamstrings and calves. This movement will also stretch your hips and lower back.

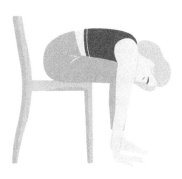

1. Begin in a seated mountain pose with your knees stacked over your ankles, hip-distance apart. Place your hands on your thighs.
2. As you inhale, lengthen your spine.
3. Exhale and slowly bend forward by hinging at your

| Seated Forward Bend

hips. Reach your hands to the feet, or if you can, to the floor. Let your head hang heavy so you can let your neck relax in the position.
4. Inhale and exhale briefly to allow your hamstrings and lower back to feel the stretch.

5. When you are ready to sit back up, inhale and slowly roll up, allowing each vertebra to stack on top of one another, with your head coming up last.

Seated Side Bends

Side bends are an excellent way to stretch your side muscles and remove any tension you may be holding there. This movement also opens your rib cage so your chest can open further. Additionally, the side bend movement can

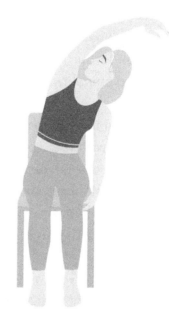

- increase your mobility and flexibility.
- strengthen your core muscles.
- improve your posture.
- improve circulation.
- improve lung capacity.

Here's how to do it:

1. Begin in a seated mountain pose with your knees stacked over your ankles, hip-distance apart. Have your arms hanging beside you.

Seated Side Bend

2. Inhale and lift your left arm overhead with your palm facing inward. Bring your right hand to the side of the chair for stability.
3. Exhale as you bend toward your right, creating a "C" shape.

4. Inhale and return to the starting position.
5. Exhale and lower your left arm to repeat the same steps on the other side.

Seated Spinal Twist

If there is one thing many yogis like to do, it's twisting! Twists help us restore and maintain our spine's range of motion. The twisting movement is significant as most of us lead a sedentary lifestyle which impacts our spine's health! Without focusing on our spine's range of motion, we allow the muscles, tendons, ligaments, and fascia to shorten and become rigid in addition to our joints fusing and hardening. Here's how to do a seated spinal twist:

1. Begin in a seated mountain pose with your knees stacked over your ankles, hip-distance apart. Ensure your back is straight.
2. To begin the twist, inhale deeply.
3. Exhale as you twist your torso to the right. Place your left hand on the outside of your right knee and your right arm on the back of your chair.

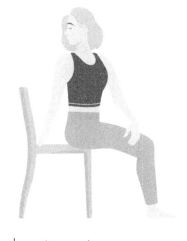

Spinal Twist

4. If you are able, with each inhale, lengthen your spine and, on the exhale, deepen the twist. Ensure you listen to your body so you are not going further than it can handle.

5. Hold for 5 to 10 breaths before untwisting your spine. Repeat on the other side.

Putting the Warmup Yoga Flow Together

To make your warmup seamless, here is how you can put the movements together:

1. Start your warmup with the sun salutation movement, feeling the energy flow through your body.
2. After you move through the sun salutation, move into doing some seated cat-cows to warm up your spine.
3. Once your spine is warmed up, move into a forward bend.
4. Next, work on warming up your sides with the side bends.
5. Finish with a spinal twist in both directions.

Cooling Down After Your Yoga Practice

Cooling down after your yoga session is just as important as warming up. They allow you to feel all of the benefits of your practice. Plus, if your yoga flow was exceptionally energizing and increased your heart rate, a cooldown will allow your heart rate to return to its resting rate, prevent muscle soreness, and improve your overall relaxed state of mind.

Seated Pigeon Pose

The pigeon pose helps support the flexibility and mobility in your hip flexors and lower back, two areas in our body that are often tight due to sitting for extended periods. You can help relieve pain or tension in your lower back and hips by stretching these muscles.

Here's how to do it:

1. Start by sitting in your chair with your butt close to the edge of the seat.
2. Place your right ankle on top of your left thigh or knee to create the shape of a four, and rest your hands on your knee.
3. Inhale to lengthen your spine.
4. On the exhale, bend at your hips to bring your chest toward your legs. Ensure that you do not round your back.
5. Stay here for a few minutes before returning to center.

Helpful tip: If you find it difficult to lift your leg to rest it on the other, use a yoga block or a stack of yoga blocks on the inside of your supporting foot and place your bent leg on top of them.

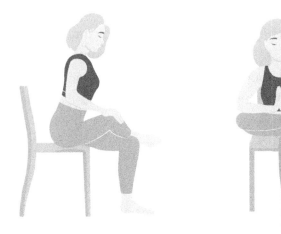

 Pigeon Pose

Alternative hands: When you can handle the pose with your hands resting on your knee, try the seated pigeon pose by holding your hands in a prayer pose as you lean further forward.

Seated Single-Leg Stretch

The seated single-leg stretch will help to stretch out your calf muscles and hamstrings. Here's how to do it:

1. Sit on your chair with your butt as close to the front as is comfortable.
2. Extend your right leg out in front of you with your toes flexed to the ceiling.
3. Inhale and bend forward to feel the stretch in your right leg. You can keep your hand resting on your shin, or if you are able to, hold your toes. Hold for a few breaths.
4. Bring your right leg back in and switch sides.

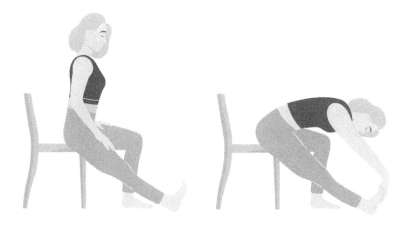

Single-Leg Stretch

Seated Child's Pose

The child's pose may not seem like it is much of anything. You may be visualizing it as the way toddlers often sleep, but it is an excellent resting pose to visit during a cooldown, or if a pose in a yoga class is too challenging for you.

However, it is more than just a resting pose. The child's pose can help to

- alleviate tension in your lower back.
- enhance blood circulation.
- aid in digestion.
- open your hips.
- stretch your shoulders.
- energize your body.
- calm the mind.

You may choose to use two chairs and a blanket or a towel for this pose. Here's how to do it:

1. Sit on your chair with the other chair across from you; with the blanket or towel folded on the seat.
2. Inhale to lengthen your spine.
3. Exhale and fold forward, resting your arms on the chair seat in front of you.

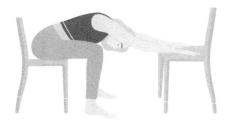

| Child's Pose With Two Chairs

You may also choose to use one chair for this pose. Here's how to do it:

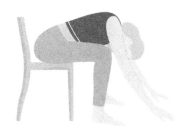

| Child's Pose

1. Exhale and fold forward, allowing your fingertips to touch the floor.
2. Stay in the position for as long as is comfortable for you.
3. When you are ready, exhale, and slowly roll back up when ready to come out of the child's pose.

Final Relaxation

At the end of your cooldown, you can end it with a seated mountain pose. You'll sit in your chair with your knees stacked over your ankles and hip-distance apart. In this position, you have multiple options on where to place your hands. You can have them resting on your thighs, in prayer position, or clasped together resting in your lap. Sit in this position for a couple of breaths as you bring your attention and focus to your body.

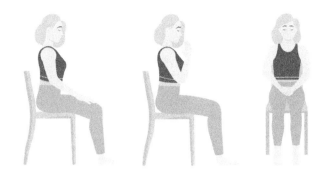

| Final Relaxation

Another movement you can include in your cooldown is the seated cat-cow to maintain your spine's posture and mobility. If you want to use this movement in the cooldown phase of your yoga session, it's best to do it before the seated pigeon pose.

Putting the Cooldown Yoga Flow Together

Remember, this cooldown can be done after your yoga practice (especially if it is a more intense practice) or after any physical activity. This is the best way to execute this flow:

1. Start your cooldown in mountain pose before moving into the seated cat-cow pose to maintain the mobility and flexibility in your spine.
2. When you are ready, extend your right leg out to do a single leg stretch.
3. After your single leg stretch, bring your right ankle across your left leg for the pigeon pose.
4. Repeat steps two to three at least four times. Once you complete the cycle on both sides, you can move into a child's pose for a few minutes.

5. Finish with the final relaxation.

Now that you know how to warm up before a yoga routine and cool down afterward, you are ready to do some yoga! The next chapter is going to cover easy chair yoga routines that are designed to improve balance.

4
Chair Yoga for Balance

Many studies are finding that yoga positively impacts balance in healthy people. As we know, balance is essential for virtually everything we do. From getting up from a lying down position, standing up from a chair, sitting down in one, and walking. But, it can become a significant problem when we get older, especially when many of us live a sedentary lifestyle. Adults who live a more active lifestyle are better prepared to react to and handle the demands of life and are more likely to avoid falls. However, regardless of which category you fit in, it's still essential to maintain your balance, range of motion, and gait to get the most out of your golden years. Chair yoga is an excellent way to improve your balance as it works on flexibility and balance training.

Balance Improving Chair Yoga Flow 1

This first chair yoga flow is designed to help you work on your balance. I find this to be a valuable flow for stretching my hips and upper body. After a long day at work, or even during the workday, I like to complete this flow to help me stretch my muscles and bring some life back into them. These poses will be done standing up using your chair for support. It should take as little as 10 minutes to complete.

Tree Pose

The tree pose, or Vrksasana, is a well-known yoga pose for yogi or non-yogi. When I think of trees, I think of the tall ones in the deeply wooded areas. They are calm, patient creatures, literally breathing life into all of us.

As a balancing yoga posture, the tree pose helps strengthen our core and legs, allowing us to open our hips and stretch the inner thigh and groin muscles. It can be pretty tricky to master, but that's where the chair will come in handy (much like baby trees having support to help them grow). Here's how to stand tall like a tree:

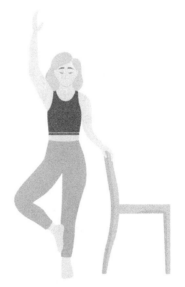

| Tree Pose

1. Stand with your right side facing the back of your chair with your right hand resting on the back.
2. Turning your left leg out, lift your heel so the balls of your feet are on the floor and your heel rests against the inside of your right leg. Picture it like a small kickstand.

3. When ready, slide your left foot up to rest entirely against your right leg just above your ankle bone or against your entire calf muscle.
4. Bring your left arm up overhead, and hold.
5. Lower and switch sides.

When you master this pose, try challenging yourself to let go of the chair and balance. You may also want to try and bring your foot to your thigh, which will make balancing a little harder as well as the stretch in your hip flexors a little deeper.

Foot-to-Seat Pose

In this foot-to-seat pose, you will have the opportunity to work on stepping motions. This movement can be challenging for seniors, especially if it is a big step! I also love this pose as it helps to stretch your hip flexors while challenging your balance. Here's how to do the exercise:

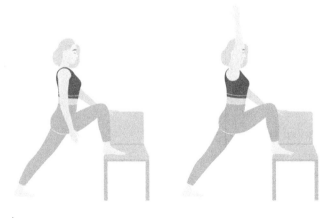

Foot-to-Seat Pose

1. Turn your chair, so it is sideways to you, and stand about two to three steps away from it.

2. Put your left hand on the back of the chair as you step your right foot onto the chair's seat. You can keep your right hand on your hip or lift your arm above your head.
3. Hold for a few moments, then switch sides.

When you master this pose, try challenging yourself to let go of the chair and balance yourself.

Triangle Pose

The triangle pose is another foundational pose. As it challenges your balance and stability, you will find that it stretches your hamstrings. Here's how to do it:

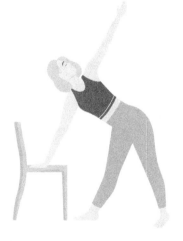

Triangle Pose

1. Place your chair so that it is sideways to you. Stand about three to four feet away from it on the left side of it with your feet hip-width apart.
2. Turn your left foot out about 45 degrees while keeping your right foot facing the chair.
3. Inhale as you raise your left arm to shoulder height.
4. Reach your right arm to the chair's seat or back on the exhale. Hold for a few moments, then repeat on the other side.

When you get stronger with this pose, you should challenge yourself further and look toward the ceiling.

Palm Tree Pose

Returning to a tree pose, we will visualize ourselves as a palm tree swaying in the warm tropical breeze this time! This pose is excellent for challenging your balance as you stand on your toes and stretch your arms, chest, core muscles, spine, and legs. Here's how to be a palm tree in yoga:

1. Stand behind your chair with your hands resting on the back.
2. Raise onto the balls of your feet.
3. As you shift your weight onto the right leg, reach your left arm overhead. You should find that the movement is similar to a side stretch.
4. Return to the center, placing your raised arm back onto the chair, and switch sides.

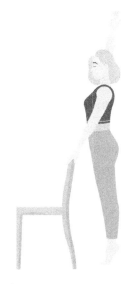

Palm Tree Pose

Putting Balance Chair Yoga Flow 1 Together

Here is how to put the first flow together:

1. Start by standing next to your chair with your right hand holding the backrest for the Tree Pose. Root your right foot into the ground and bend your left knee, placing the sole of your left foot on the inside of your right leg. You can choose whether it feels better on your ankle, calf, or above the knee, but make sure it's not directly on the knee. Raise your left arm overhead

once your foot is in a comfortable spot, and balance here for a few breaths.

2. Gently lower your left foot to the ground while holding onto the chair for support. Then, transition yourself so the chair is sideways to you with your left hand resting on the back for the Foot-to-Seat Pose. Standing about two to three steps away from the chair, step your right foot onto the chair's seat. Place your right hand on your hip or lift your arm above your head for an additional challenge, and balance here for a few breaths before transitioning to the Triangle Pose.

3. Place your right foot back on the ground while holding onto the chair with your left hand. Facing the front of your chair, place your feet shoulder-width apart, with your left foot pointing towards the chair and your right foot facing forward. Shift your right hip back, slide your left hand down the chair, and extend your right arm towards the ceiling. This should create a nice straight line from your left hand to your right. Remember to keep both legs straight and your chest open. Hold this pose for a few breaths and then rise back up.

4. Returning to face the back of your chair with your feet together, rest your hands on the back for the Palm Tree Pose. As you inhale, raise onto the balls of your feet. As you exhale, shift your weight onto the right leg and reach your left arm overhead. Lift your left heel off the floor to feel a nice side stretch. Inhale to move back to the center, placing your raised arm back onto the chair to switch sides. Keep swaying side to side like a palm tree in the breeze for a few breaths.

5. Repeat this sequence on the other side.

Balance Improving Chair Yoga Flow 2

Similar to the first flow, this is an excellent way to bring energy back into our legs after a long day of sitting. It's especially helpful to engage our leg muscles before we start any activity that could be a little more strenuous, which could be something as simple as cleaning the house. Think of it as a warmup to what we're doing next.

Chair Staff Pose

The chair staff pose is a foundational seated pose equivalent to a seated mountain pose except that you have your legs extended out in front of you. This pose helps to stretch your calves and hamstrings while boosting spinal awareness. Here's how to do it:

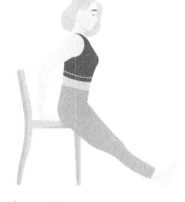

Staff Pose

1. Sit close to the edge of your chair with your feet extended out in front of you and your toes pointed to the ceiling.
2. Place your hands behind your butt on the seat with your fingers facing the front.
3. Push into your hands to gently push your upper body forward until you feel a stretch in your calves and hamstrings. Hold for a few moments, and then release.

Chair Bound Angle Pose

The bound angle pose is a variation of the butterfly pose, and it is excellent to help strengthen and improve the flexibility in your thighs, knees, and groins. It's also a pose that can help relieve the symptoms associated with sciatica and lower back pain. For this yoga pose, I'd recommend using a couple of yoga blocks or a rolled-up pillow to support your ankles. Here's how to do it:

1. Sit close to the edge of your chair with your yoga blocks stacked in front of you. Your hands can rest on the seat or your thighs.
2. Rest the outside of your ankles on the block, allowing your knees to flop open. Try to get the bottoms of your feet touching it if you can.
3. Hold the pose for one minute.

For an added challenge, you can use a second chair in place of the yoga blocks. Here's how to do it:

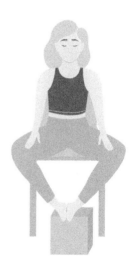

Bound Angle Pose With Yoga Blocks

1. Sit close to the edge of your chair with the other chair facing you. Your hands can rest on the seat or your thighs, or you may place them in the prayer position.
2. Rest the outside of your ankles on the edge of the second chair, allowing your knees fall to the side. Try to get the bottoms of your feet touching it if you can.

Also, in this flow, include the forward bend and seated pigeon pose as previously described in Chapter 3.

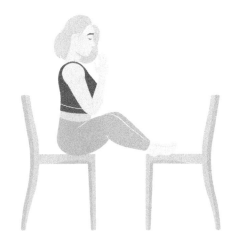

| Bound Angle Pose

Putting Balance Chair Yoga Flow 2 Together

If you want to put together this second flow, here is how to do it:

1. First, sit comfortably on your chair, feet planted firmly on the ground, about hip distance apart for a forward bend. On a big inhale, reach your arms up towards the sky, lengthening your spine. As you exhale, fold forward from your hips, letting your hands rest on your shins, ankles, or the floor, depending on your flexibility. Let your head hang down for a few breaths before moving into the staff pose.

2. Slowly roll your body up, one vertebra at a time, until you're sitting tall again. Once you're sitting upright, extend your legs straight out in front of you, keeping

your feet flexed and active. Place your hands behind your butt on the seat with your fingers facing the front and push into your hands to gently push your upper body forward until you feel a stretch in your calves and hamstrings.

3. To move into the pigeon pose, bend your right knee to place your right foot flat on the ground. Then, place your left ankle over your right knee, creating a figure-four shape with your legs. If this feels good, you can stay here. If you want a deeper stretch, gently lean forward from your hips. You should feel this in your left hip for a great stretch and balance challenge.

4. After a few breaths in pigeon pose, gently uncross your leg, returning your foot to the floor. Scoot forward slightly on your chair so that there's room for your feet to come together. Bring the soles of your feet together on your yoga block or chair, and let your knees drop to the sides. Hold for a couple of breaths.

5. Switch sides and repeat steps one through four.

Balance Improving Chair Yoga Flow 3

In this 10-minute chair yoga flow, your balance is tested through various poses! This is another full-body workout flow as it engages multiple parts of our body. I enjoy this flow for a couple of other reasons as well. First, this flow requires a bit more mental concentration as we focus on our balance moving between positions. As a result, this is a great option for a morning flow as it helps our bodies and minds wake up. Second (and most importantly, in my opinion), this is an empowering flow. Not only because of the message the

Warrior poses tells us but since it requires more concentration, I walk away from the flow feeling accomplished.

Warrior I Pose

The Warrior is an interesting character and symbol in so many cultures! However, this pose (and the upcoming three Warrior poses) have a sense of empowerment through each movement.

The Warrior I pose strengthens your legs as you open your chest and hips and stretch your arms and legs. This pose also helps to improve your circulation and your respiration. As you stand in this pose, feel the energy that flows through you as you root yourself to the Earth.

1. Begin by sitting in your chair in mountain pose.
2. Turn to the right to sit sideways on your chair.
3. Keeping your right foot facing the front, extend your left leg to the side, aiming to keep your left foot on the floor with your hips facing the right.
4. Take a deep inhale and lift both arms above your head with your palms facing in.
5. On the exhale, shift your left leg behind you as far as is comfortable.

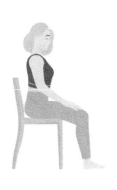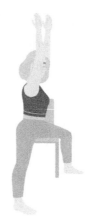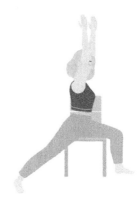

| Warrior I Pose

Warrior II Pose

Warrior II takes the foundational Warrior pose to the next level, bringing power, strength, and vision as you root yourself to the Earth. Beyond its symbolic nature, Warrior II helps to create flexibility in your hips and legs. You can continue into this pose from Warrior I. Here's how to do Warrior II:

1. From Warrior I on the right side, inhale as you turn your torso toward the front of your chair.
2. Exhale and bring your arms down until they are shoulder height with your palms facing the floor.

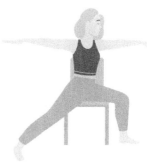

| Warrior II Pose

Reverse Warrior Pose

The reverse Warrior pose helps to strengthen your legs as you open the side of your body from a side bend and improve the mobility in your spine along with your core and balance strength. This pose is also very energizing as it supports your respiration and circulation throughout your body. You can flow into this move from Warrior II.

1. From Warrior II, allow your left arm to come down behind you.
2. Inhale and bring your right arm toward the ceiling as you bend sideways. Rest your left hand on your left leg for support.
3. To return to the starting position. Bring your legs back in and turn to sit on the front of your chair to return to the seated mountain pose.

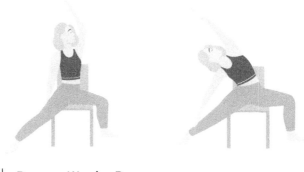

Reverse Warrior Pose

Chair-Supported Upward Facing Dog

The chair-supported upward facing dog is an active pose that energizes your upper body strength and strengthens your wrists, arms, and core muscles while alleviating pain and discomfort in your lower back. Here's how to do it:

1. Place your chair in front of you and against a wall to prevent it from moving. Alternatively, you can place your chair on a yoga mat.
2. Bend forward and place your hands on your chair to hold the edges.
3. Step back until your body is about 45 degrees from the ground. Ensure you curl your toes under to feel a stretch of your calves.

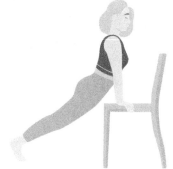

4. As you inhale, lift your chest until you have a slight bend in your back.

| Upward Facing Dog

5. Exhale to deepen the backbend as far as is comfortable for you. On your last inhale, release the pose and step forward to come out of it.

Chair-Supported Downward Facing Dog

The downward facing dog pose is another well-known yoga pose, even if you aren't a seasoned yogi. It can help you build bone density as you place weight through your shoulders and arms and can help revitalize your energy if you're feeling fatigued. This pose will be done with the support of your chair. You have a couple of options for how you use your chair. You can use the chair seat for support, or if you need something higher or additional support, use the backrest instead. Here's how to do it:

1. Stand in front of or behind your chair and lean down to rest your hands on the chair seat or backrest.

2. Take a few steps back from the chair. Ensure your spine is straight and your feet are hip-width apart.

3. As you press your hand into the chair, roll your shoulders back and down away from your ears. Stay here and breathe deeply for three to five breaths.

4. On your last inhale, step back toward your chair and slowly roll up to a standing position.

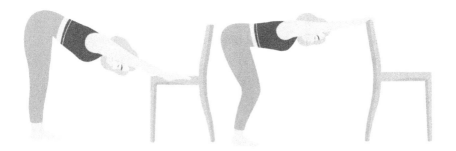

| Downward Facing Dog

Putting Balance Chair Yoga Flow 3 Together

For the last flow, here is how you can put all of the moves together to become a Warrior of yoga:

1. We'll kick things off with seated warrior I. Sit up nice and tall on the edge of your chair. Rotate to the right so your right leg is bent over the side of the chair and your right foot is flat on the floor. Extend your left leg behind you, toes pointed back, and resting on the ground. Sweep your arms up towards the sky and take a moment to find your balance.

2. While maintaining your leg positions, simply rotate your upper body to the left, lowering your arms to the sides at shoulder height, your right arm pointing

forward, and your left arm pointing back for
warrior II.

3. Keeping your legs as they are, drop your left arm down
    to rest on the back of your left leg and reach your
    right arm up towards the sky for reverse warrior,
    creating a nice stretch on your right side. Remember
    to keep that right knee bent and hold your balance.

4. To move into downward facing dog, bring your right
    arm back down, pivot your body back to the front of
    the chair to stand up. Place your chair in front of you
    (either on a yoga mat or against a wall to prevent it
    from moving) and take two to three steps back before
    bending forward at the hips to place your hands on
    the seat about shoulder-width apart to form a nice "V"
    shape with your hips being the highest point. Press
    your palms into the chair, draw your belly in, and push
    your hips back. Your head should be in line with your
    arms. Hold for two more breaths.

5. On your last exhale, simultaneously lower your hips
    and lift your chest until your body is about 45 degrees
    from the ground for the upward facing dog. Once you
    feel sturdy, inhale and lift your chest until you have a
    slight bend in your back and exhale to deepen the
    backbend to your comfort level. On your last exhale,
    slowly reverse the pose to pass through downward
    facing dog before slowly rolling up to a standing
    position. Then switch sides and repeat.

Yoga has not only been shown to improve your balance, but it
can help relieve joint and arthritic pain as well. In the next
chapter, you will discover some simple yoga routines
designed to alleviate joint pain.

The Ripple Effect

Let's take a moment and breathe. You've made it to the heart of this transformative journey. As you dive deeper into the pages of the book, I want to take a moment to remind you of the incredible impact you can have on others.

You see, the power of this book lies not only in the wisdom it imparts but in the community it fosters. Each and every word you read is an invitation to connect, not just with yourself, but with countless others who are on their own unique paths toward wellness. So, I encourage you to share your journey. Don't keep it to yourself when you reach a moment of break-through or a realization that resonates deeply. The power of connection lies in our ability to share and support one another.

Imagine the lives you can touch by sharing your experience. As you learn and grow through the practice of chair yoga, think about the individuals who might be seeking a similar transformation. Your words have the power to inspire, ignite a spark within someone's heart, and guide them toward a life filled with greater independence, vitality, and joy.

I encourage you to commit to yourself and those who may benefit from your journey. When you reach the end of this book, take a moment to reflect on the impact it has had on your life. Then, summon the courage to share your story by writing a review, not just for the book but for potential readers who are still on the fence. Your honest feedback can help them make an informed decision and take that first step towards a healthier and more fulfilling life. Let your words serve as a beacon of hope, guiding them toward the transformative benefits of chair yoga.

You can also share your experiences with friends, family, or even your local community. Invite others to join you on this wonderful journey and witness its positive impact on their lives. By creating space for others to experience yoga's healing and empowering effects, you become an agent of change and a source of inspiration.

Remember, the ripple effect of your actions can extend far beyond what you can imagine. By sharing your story, you have the power to touch lives, uplift spirits, and ignite a passion for wellness in others. Your words, whether spoken or written, can create a ripple that spreads joy, healing, and transformation throughout your community.

So, my dear reader, embrace the opportunity to give back. Together, we can create a world where chair yoga is accessible to all and where each person's unique journey contributes to the well-being of others.

Thank you for being a part of this beautiful community. Your willingness to share and support is what makes it thrive. Keep shining your light, and let your words inspire others to embark on their own transformative chair yoga adventure.

5

Chair Yoga for Joint and Arthritic Pain

Let's be honest: Joint paint is very uncomfortable, especially when it involves arthritis. According to the Cleveland Clinic, "arthritis is the most common cause of disability" in the United States, where around "50 million adults" have some form of arthritis. Different types of arthritis have varying causes, including:

- family history.
- jobs or sports that put consistent stress on your joints.
- autoimmune diseases or viral infections.

The good news is recent clinical studies are finding that yoga can be a therapeutic way to manage arthritis. For example, in 2018, a meta-analysis of 1,557 patients with knee osteoarthritis and rheumatoid arthritis participated in 13 clinical trials. These studies found that yoga may help reduce the symptoms associated with knee arthritis and enhance both physical function and the general well-being of arthritic patients.

Everyone should be exercising—that much we know. However, physical activity is especially important for people with arthritis, as a lack of movement will lead to a loss of muscle strength, endurance, and physical energy. In addition, living with arthritis tends to make you more sedentary, as moving your joints hurts. It's understandable, but not moving impairs your range of motion which in turn makes the pain worse, and repeat—it's a painful hamster wheel to be on. So how do you get off the hamster wheel of pain? Chair yoga, my friend!

Chair yoga puts less stress on your joints; you can work on alleviating some of the pain associated with arthritis or other joint pain. It's one way to gently ease your joints into movement while maintaining endurance and muscle strength. Plus, easing your joints into stretching movements will do wonders for them.

But it's not just about the physical relief that chair yoga can provide your aches and pains. Chair yoga has various psychological advantages, especially when your joints are hurting and are causing you stress as a result. In addition, decreasing stress and depressive symptoms through yoga helps boost general well-being and immune function—which are very important for those with arthritis.

Routine for Easing Arthritis Pain

As we talked about earlier, one of the best remedies for arthritis is movement so we can prevent muscle loss and stiff joints. This flow is perfect as it works most joints throughout our bodies. This is an excellent flow to keep in your back pocket, and pull it out about once a week to keep those joints fresh.

In this first yoga routine to ease joint pain, we will reuse some poses we have seen in previous chapters. Therefore the following poses will not include instructions:

- Warrior II (Chapter 4)
- Seated spinal twist and seated cat-cow pose (Chapter 3)

Reverse Chair Pose

In general, the chair pose benefits us all as the movement engages our legs, upper and lower back, shoulders, hamstrings, glutes, hips, and feet. This yoga pose is excellent for elongating your back to strengthen your core muscles while relieving stiffness in your arms, legs, shoulders, and back.

Typically, this pose is done from a standing position when an instructor has the class perform a root-to-rise. However, with your chair, you'll begin from a seated position. Here's how to do it:

1. Sit in your chair in mountain pose, with your bottom as close to the edge as is comfortable. Rest your hands on your thighs.
2. Inhale and lift your arms above your head with your palms facing each other and fingers pointed to the ceiling.

3. Exhale and push your weight through your heels to stand up partially from your chair. Your ending pose should be a high squat where your legs are about 45 degrees. Make sure your spine remains straight with your neck in line with it.
4. Hold for three to five breaths and then slowly lower back to your chair to return to mountain pose.

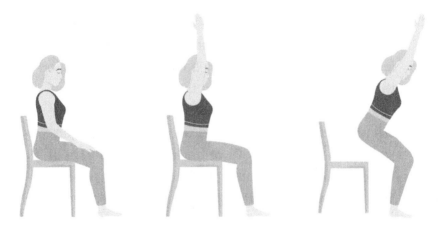

Reverse Chair Pose

Putting the Arthritis Flow Together

Now that you know how to execute the exercises, here is how to put everything together in a seamless flow:

1. Start by sitting up tall toward the edge of your chair with your feet flat on the floor and your hands on your thighs. As you inhale, arch your back and push your chest out for the cow pose. As you exhale, round your back, pull your belly in, and let your head drop forward for the cat pose. Keep flowing between these two

poses, syncing with your breath. From the cat pose, gently come back to a neutral seated position.

2. Sit up tall for the spinal twist pose, and as you exhale, twist your upper body to the right, placing your right hand on the back of the chair and your left hand on your right knee. Look over your right shoulder, hold for a few breaths, then inhale to return to the center.

3. From the center, rotate to the right so that your right leg is bent over the side of the chair and your right foot is flat on the floor for Warrior II. Extend your left leg behind you, toes pointing backward and resting on the floor. Extend your arms to the sides at shoulder height, with your right arm pointing forward and your left arm pointing back, gazing over your right fingers. Hold for a few breaths. Pivot back to face the front of the chair with both feet back on the ground.

4. To move into the reverse chair pose, scoot a bit to the edge of your chair, keeping your feet flat on the floor, hip-distance apart. On an inhale, lift your arms overhead with your palms facing each other and fingers pointed to the ceiling. As you exhale, keep your spine straight and push your weight through your heels to stand up partially from your chair until your legs are at about 45 degrees. Hold here for about three to five breaths before slowly lowering back to your chair to return to a mountain pose.

5. Repeat steps two through four, twisting to the left for your spinal twist and putting your left leg in from when you reach Warrior II.

Routine for Easing Hip Pain

This routine is one of my favorites! I work in front of a computer all day, so I sit at my desk for eight to nine hours a day. By the time the afternoon rolls around, my hips are starting to ache. So, I'll take a quick pause and move through this flow. Not only does it help ease my aches, but I typically get a little boost of energy as well.

When I think of our hips, they are the secondary supporting factor for our body (next to our legs). So when our hips hurt, it makes walking a difficult feat (no pun intended).

Thankfully, yoga can help hip pain by strengthening and stabilizing the joint while stretching and lengthening the surrounding ligaments and tendons.

This yoga routine will use poses to help our hips with pain, mobility, and flexibility. As done in the previous section, some poses of earlier chapters will be re-used, and the instructions will not be included in this section:

- Seated bound angle pose (Chapter 4)
- Seated pigeon pose (Chapter 3)

Seated Hip Circles

As the name suggests, seated hip circles involve moving your hips in a circular motion while seated in your chair. It's similar to pelvic circles, which you would do from a standing position.

Here's how to do it:

1. Sit in your chair with a tall spine and your hands on your thighs or knees.
2. Begin to make slow circular motions with your torso at your hips in a clockwise rotation.
3. As you continue to rotate, allow your circles to become larger.
4. After at least five rotations, return to the center and repeat in a counterclockwise rotation.

Seated Half-Wind Relieving Pose

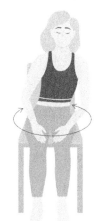

The wind-relieving pose is exactly as it sounds: It can help to release gas pent up in your abdomen. However, it can also help to relieve stress and pain in your hips by stretching your hamstrings.

Seated Hip
Circles

1. Sit in your chair with your legs about hip-distance apart.
2. Lift your right leg and clasp your fingers behind your knee to pull your leg in closer to your chest.
3. Hold for a few breaths, then release.
4. Repeat on the other side.

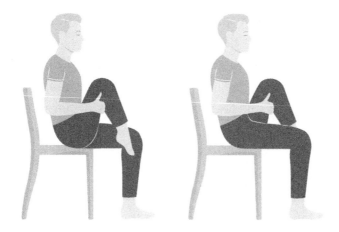

Half Wind Relieving pose

Putting the Hip Pain Flow Together

Here is how to put these four moves together:

1. Start with hip circles by sitting up tall on your chair with your feet flat on the floor and your hands resting on your knees or thighs. Imagine sitting on a giant clock and trying to move your hips to every number, making big circles in a clockwise rotation. As you continue to rotate, allow your circles to become larger. After five rotations, return to the center and repeat counterclockwise. After your last hip circle, return to a neutral sitting position to prepare for deep hip stretches.

2. Make sure your feet are flat on the floor, and your legs are hip-distance apart, lift your right foot off the floor, and bring your right knee towards your chest for the half wind relieving pose. Clasp your fingers behind your knee to pull your leg closer to your chest. Hold this pose for a few breaths, feeling a gentle stretch in

your right hip. When ready, release and return your right foot to the floor.

3. Move into the pigeon pose by placing your right ankle over your left knee, creating a figure-four shape with your legs. If this feels good, you can stay here. If you want a deeper stretch, gently lean forward from your hips. You should feel this in your right hip for a great stretch and balance challenge.

4. After a few breaths in pigeon pose, gently uncross your leg, returning your foot to the floor. Scoot forward slightly on your chair so that there's room for your feet to come together. Bring the soles of your feet together on your yoga block or chair and let your knees drop to the sides. Hold the bound angle pose for a couple of breaths.

5. Repeat steps two through four, focusing on your left side for the seated half-wind relieving pose and the seated pigeon pose.

Routine for Easing Joint Pain

I use this flow when I want to focus on opening my hips and chest, especially when my shoulders are acting up. Again, I love that I can perform this yoga flow right from my desk at work. But also at the dinner table or even on the couch. The couch is probably where I use this the most and it's in the morning while I'm still waking up. This is a great way to ease into a busy day.

Waking up in the morning with stiff joints is not an ideal motivator to get up from bed. However, this flow can help build range of motion to help you start your day off on the right foot.

In this flow, we will reuse downward facing dog. If you need a refresher on how to execute the pose, refer back to Chapter 4.

Seated Goddess Pose

Like the Warrior, a goddess is a very powerful symbol in Indian mythology, representing everything that makes up our universe. This first goddess pose we will be using in this flow helps us

- open our hips, legs, and chest.
- strengthen our legs and shoulders.
- stretches the shoulder joint and chest muscles.

It's not a widely used pose in traditional yoga, but to help ease your joints, it can do a lot. Here is how to do it:

1. Sit on your chair in mountain pose with a straight spine and your hands resting on your thighs.
2. On your inhale, open your legs to a wide stance, ensuring your knees remain stacked over your ankles and your toes are pointed outward. Lift your arms above your head.
3. Exhale and bend your elbows to create cactus arms.
4. Hold for a few moments.

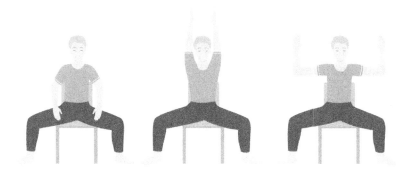

Seated Goddess Pose

Seated Goddess Pose With a Twist

This twisting pose has an added level as your legs will be widened. This added element will help your hips stretch as you twist. In addition, this pose will help release any tension your spine may be holding. Here is how to do it:

1. Sit on your chair in mountain pose with a straight spine and your hands resting on your thighs.
2. On your inhale, open your legs to a wide stance, ensuring your knees remain stacked over your ankles and your toes are pointed outward.
3. Exhale as you twist your body to the right, grabbing the back of your chair with your right arm and resting your left hand on the outside of your right thigh. Hold for a few moments, then slowly untwist.
4. Repeat on the other side.

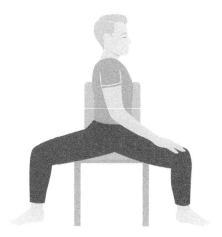

| Goddess Pose With a Twist

Seated Goddess Pose With a Side Bend

Adding a side bend to your seated goddess pose will help lengthen your hip joint and side muscles and release shoulder pain. This pose is also going to help you open your chest muscles. Here is how to do it:

1. Sit on your chair in mountain pose with a straight spine and your hands resting on your thighs.
2. On your inhale, open your legs to a wide stance, ensuring your knees remain stacked over your ankles and your toes are pointed outward.
3. Bring your hands behind your head.
4. Exhale as you lean sideways to the right, pointing your right elbow to the floor.
5. Inhale to come back to the center.
6. Repeat on the other side.

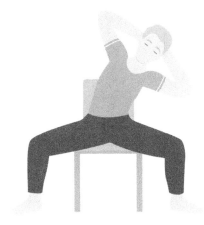

| Seated Goddess Pose With A Side Bend

Seated Goddess Pose Forward Bend

This final goddess pose in this flow will bring restoration into your body. It will stretch your hips, groin, inner thighs, and back while strengthening your shoulders, lower back, and knees. This movement is excellent for those who cannot bend over due to limitations, as you only need to have your hands resting on your thighs.

1. Sit in your chair with your legs widened and your toes facing outward.
2. With your hands on your inner thighs, inhale to engage your core muscles.
3. Slowly lean forward until your spine is on a diagonal.
4. Hold for a few moments, then slowly sit back up to an upright position.

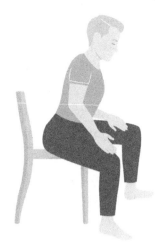

Seated Goddess Pose Forward
Fold

Putting the Joint Pain Flow Together

Here is how to put this final flow together for joint pain:

1. Let's start with the goddess pose by sitting on the
   edge of your chair in mountain pose with a straight
   spine and your hands resting on your thighs. On your
   inhale, open your legs to a wide stance, turning your
   toes outward and ensuring your knees remain stacked
   over your ankles. Raise your arms over your head with
   your palms facing each other and your fingers
   pointing to the sky. Then, bend your elbows to 90
   degrees, palms facing forward, to create cactus arms.
2. While maintaining your goddess's legs, let's add a
   side bend to the mix. Bring your hands behind your
   head, interlocking your fingers. Exhale as you lead
   your torso sideways to the right, pointing your right
   elbow to the floor, feeling the stretch along your left

side. After a few breaths, return to the center and bring your hands to your thighs.

3. Move your hands to your inner thighs and inhale to engage your core muscles. As you exhale, fold your upper body between your knees, ensuring your neck and spine remain straight and connected. Remember to listen to your body and only bend forward as far as what makes sense for you. Hang out here for a few breaths, releasing tension in your lower back and hips. Slowly lift your torso to the seated goddess pose, and let's move into a twist.

4. From the center, exhale as you twist your body to the right, grabbing the back of your chair with your right arm and resting your left hand on the outside of your right thigh. Hold here for a few moments before you slowly untwist.

5. Carefully come back to a neutral seated position, stand up from your chair, and turn so that you are facing the chair seat for the downward facing dog pose. Bend your torso toward the chair seat and take a couple of steps forward until your body forms a nice "V" shape, with your hips being the highest point. Press your palms into the chair, draw your belly in, and push your hips back. Your head should be in line with your arms. On your last inhale, step toward your chair and slowly roll up to a standing position.

6. Repeat steps two to five, focusing on the left side.

In addition to relieving joint pain, evidence has shown that practicing yoga can improve mobility in people overall. In the next chapter, you will discover several easy chair yoga routines that are designed to improve mobility.

6
Chair Yoga for Mobility

How does back pain impact our lifestyle? Most of us have dealt with back pain at some point or another. We could have caused a lower back spasm from a simple movement, such as picking up something from the floor, or the spasm could be the starting factor to a more significant issue like a bulged or herniated disc. Big or small, back pain, and lower back pain, more specifically, impact our quality of life when the pain flares up and stays there longer than it should. Unfortunately, back pain's unwelcome stay is the "leading cause of activity limitation and work absence throughout much of the world" (Hoy et al., 2014).

While basic stretching is recommended for people with impacted mobility due to lower back pain, yoga, as another activity, is just as good to help reduce lower back pain. In fact, according to John Hopkins Medicine, "The American College of Physicians recommends yoga as a first-line treatment for chronic low back pain" (9 Benefits of Yoga, n.d.).

Back pain, and any other type of pain that impacts your mobility, is not convenient, but it also shouldn't be the factor that stops you from doing the activities you love. Most, if not all, yoga practices involve a holistic approach to improve your flexibility, balance, and strength, which all factor into having excellent mobility. I hope you have begun to understand how impactful yoga can be in your life, as we are about halfway through this journey together. That said, this chapter will look at three types of yoga flows you can incorporate into a 10-minute spot in your day to help improve overall mobility.

Routine for Increased Mobility 1

This is another routine I'll use in the morning to help release the tension from sleeping and wake my muscles. Sometimes I don't even get out of bed! I'll sit in bed in a bound-angle pose and move through the flow.

In this first chair yoga flow, we will include some exercises we've done in previous chapters and add some new ones. The exercises we will be reusing are seated yoga side bends, seated spinal twists, and seated single-leg stretches from Chapter 3.

Head Circles

Of the many places we can hold stress in our bodies, our necks seem to get the brunt! Unfortunately, it can be painful to turn our heads when we have a stiff neck. Therefore, the head circles exercise will help to relieve stiffness as you work to get the range of motion back into your neck.

1. Sit in your chair with your hands resting on your thighs or knees and a tall spine. Take a long, slow inhale.
2. On the exhale, start to make a slow circle with your head in a clockwise position. For a visual: Imagine your nose is pointing at a clock. Begin at the 12 o'clock position and circle your head around as if your nose is rotating between the minutes and hours on the clock.
3. After five rotations, change directions to circle your head counterclockwise, ensuring you begin with a long inhale.

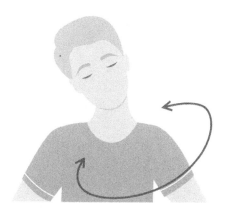

| Head Circles

Shoulder Rolls

Our shoulders are another area we tend to hold stress. Additionally, if you are a side sleeper, you may tense one of your shoulders up to your ears (and you may not even realize it). Shoulder rolls help to return the range of motion to your shoulder joints and muscles. Even without tense shoulders, they feel great to do every once in a while during the day!

1. Sit tall in your chair with your hands resting on your thighs or knees.
2. Lift your shoulders toward your ear and down to create one rotation. Continue the same movement until you reach 10 shoulder rolls, gradually making the rolls bigger as you go (you may end up lifting your arms into chicken wings).
3. Switch directions, following the same steps with your shoulders going forward.

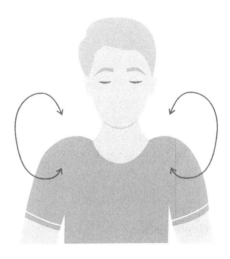

| Shoulder Rolls

Putting Increased Mobility 1 Together

This simple routine is one you may want to do when you wake up in the morning to boost the range of mobility throughout your upper body and hips.

1. Start with some head circles by sitting comfortably with your feet flat on the floor and your hands resting on your thighs or knees with a tall spine. Take a long, slow inhale. On the exhale, drop your chin to your chest and slowly roll your head clockwise in a big circle, letting it drop back, then to the right, forward, and left. Do this a few times in both directions. Be deliberate in your motions to ensure your neck is well cared for. Bring your head back up to a neutral position.

2. Moving to shoulder rolls, lift your shoulders towards your ears, then roll them back, down, and forward in a circular motion. Start with small rotations and gradually move into larger ones, then switch direction. This is such a simple way to loosen up those tight shoulder joints.

3. After your last shoulder roll, let your shoulders relax and place your arms beside you. Inhale and raise your left arm overhead with your palm facing inward for a seated side bend. Bring your right hand to the side of the chair for stability—exhale as you bend toward your right, creating a "C" shape. You'll feel a nice stretch along your left side. After a few breaths, return to the center and bring your left arm down to prepare for a spinal twist.

4. Adjust your arms by placing your left hand on your right knee and your right hand on the back of your chair. Inhale deeply and, as you exhale, twist your upper body to the right. Make sure your spine remains tall as you hold for a few breaths. Inhale to come back to the center for the single-leg stretch.

5. Scoot your butt as close to the front as is comfortable. Extend your left leg straight out in front of you with your toes flexed to the ceiling. Inhale and bend forward to feel the stretch in your left hamstring. Reach your hands towards your left foot resting on your shin. If you can touch your foot, great! If not, no worries. Listening to your body and reaching as far as feels good is more important. After a few breaths, release and return to the center.
6. Repeat steps four through six on the right side.

Routine for Increased Mobility 2

This flow is perfect for incorporating into your daily routine and can be done at any time of the day. However, I personally find that this sequence works best for me after a long walk. I use it as a cooldown, as it helps me stretch my legs and back.

In this routine, we will learn a new pose while using a variety of yoga poses we have already learned to further improve the mobility in your spine and upper back. These exercises include:

- shoulder rolls
- forward bend (Chapter 3)
- seated spinal twist (Chapter 3)
- seated single leg stretch (Chapter 3)

Seated Eagle Pose

The eagle pose, whether standing or sitting, has all the benefits you'd look for in a yoga pose: strength, flexibility, and balance. However, it also has holistic benefits to encourage a boosted immune system.

Our bodies always look for good circulation, which is crucial for good immunity. Our immune cells are always ready for anything invasive they may need to fight off. When our circulation is hindered, it impairs the ability of the immune cells to move easily. In the eagle pose, your arms will twist up into themselves, narrowing the blood flow throughout your body. As you unfurl your arms, you can revitalize the circulation to help the immune cells continue their quest to protect you.

In terms of how the eagle pose can help your arms, shoulders, and back with flexibility, your shoulders and upper back will be able to loosen in the pose, removing any stiffness you may be feeling. In addition, if you cross your legs, you can strengthen your inner thighs, as well, to improve your balance! Here's how to do it:

1. Sit in your chair in mountain pose.
2. If you can, cross your right leg over your left and tuck your right foot behind your left calf. If neither of those is possible for you, keep your legs in mountain pose with your feet hip-width apart.
3. Hug yourself by crossing your arms across your chest and touching the opposite shoulders with your right arm on top.
4. If you can, lift the back of your hands to meet each other in front of your face. If you can go further, tuck your left hand so your fingers touch your right palm. Lift your elbows to deepen the stretch and remain there for a few breaths, maintaining a good posture in your spine.

5. Release and switch sides.

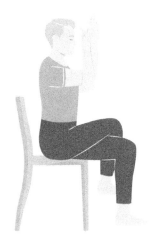

Seated Eagle Pose

Putting Increased Mobility 2 Together

1. Let's begin with your eyes closed in mountain pose, sitting comfortably on your chair with your feet flat on the floor, shoulder-width apart, and your hands resting on your thighs or knees. Sit up tall and roll your shoulders back, opening your chest. Inhale to engage your core and lift your spine. As you exhale, bring one hand to your heart and the other to your belly and imagine your body is rooting itself on the ground.

2. Moving to shoulder rolls, lift your shoulders towards your ears, then roll them back, down, and forward in a circular motion. Start with small rotations and gradually move into larger ones, then switch direction.

3. Then, inhale and reach your arms towards the sky, lengthening your spine. As you exhale, fold forward

from your hips, letting your hands rest on your shins, ankles, or the floor, depending on your flexibility. Let your head hang down for a few breaths, feeling the gentle stretch in your back. When ready, roll your body back up to seated mountain pose.

4. Scoot your butt as close to the front as is comfortable. Extend your left leg straight out in front of you with your toes flexed to the ceiling. Inhale and bend forward to feel the stretch in your left hamstring. Reach your hands towards your left foot resting on your shin. If you can touch your foot, great! If not, no worries. Listening to your body and reaching as far as feels good is more important. After a few breaths, release and return to the center.

5. Move into eagle pose by crossing your arms across your chest and touching the opposite shoulders with your right arm on top. Lift the back of your hands to meet each other in front of your face. If you want to go further, tuck your left hand so your fingers touch your right palm. Lift your elbows to deepen the stretch and remain here for a few breaths, maintaining your posture. Slowly unwind your arms and let them rest in your lap before moving into a spinal twist.

6. Inhale as you place your left hand on your right knee and your right hand on the back of your chair. As you exhale, twist your torso to the right, gazing over your right shoulder. Breathe deeply here for a few moments, then inhale to return to the center.

7. Repeat steps two through five, focusing on your left side for the seated eagle pose and seated spinal twist.

Routine for Increased Mobility 3

In this final routine to increase mobility, we will revisit some of my favorite poses, including:

- sun salutations (Chapter 3)
- seated cat-cow pose (Chapter 3)
- seated-half wind relieving pose (Chapter 5)
- reverse chair pose (Chapter 5)
- chair-supported downward facing dog pose (Chapter 4)

This routine is excellent for mid-day relief, post-workout, or even winding down before bed.

Putting Increased Mobility 3 Together

1. Let's start by sitting comfortably in your chair, feet planted firmly on the ground as we flow through the seated sun salutation. Begin in a seated mountain pose with your knees stacked over your ankles, hip-distance apart. As you inhale deeply, lift your arms over your head, stretching them toward the sky. Exhale into a prayer pose as you bring your hands to your heart center. Keeping your hands in the same position, fold forward by hinging at your hips and rounding your spine. Release your hands, reaching them toward your feet. Inhale and roll up, imagining your vertebrae stacking on one another with your head lifting last. Lastly, roll your shoulders so they are

pulled away from your ears, and rest your hands on your thighs.

2. Place your hands on your thighs for the seated cat-cow pose. As you inhale, arch your back and roll your shoulders down, lifting your chest and gazing upwards for cow pose. As you exhale, round your spine, tuck your chin, and let your shoulders and head come forward for cat pose. Continue to flow between these two poses a few times, linking your breath with the movement. After your last round of cat-cow, take a moment to come back to a neutral spine.

3. Make sure your feet are flat on the floor, and your legs are hip-distance apart, lift your right foot off the floor, and bring your right knee towards your chest for the half wind relieving pose. Clasp your fingers behind your knee to pull your leg closer to your chest. Hold this pose for a few breaths, feeling a gentle stretch in your right hip. When ready, release and return your right foot to the floor before switching sides.

4. Slide to the edge of your chair, keeping your feet flat on the floor, hip-distance apart for the reverse chair pose. On an inhale, lift your arms overhead with your palms facing each other, and fingers pointed to the ceiling. As you exhale, keep your spine straight and push your weight through your heels to stand up partially from your chair until your legs are at about 45 degrees. Hold here for about three to five breaths before slowly lowering back to your chair to return to a mountain pose. Lift your arms again to repeat the reverse chair, pushing your weight through your heels to lift yourself into the chair pose. This time, after

three to five breaths, straighten your spine to a standing mountain pose.

5. Once standing, turn to face your chair for downward facing dog. Bend your torso toward the seat of the chair and take a couple of steps forward until your body forms a nice "V" shape, with your hips being the highest point. Press your palms into the chair, draw your belly in, and push your hips back. Your head should be in line with your arms. On your last inhale, step toward your chair and slowly roll up to a standing position.

6. Repeat the flow one to three more times for a more challenging workout.

Chair yoga not only improves your range of motion, but it can be great for building strength as well. The next chapter will contain several great strength-building chair yoga routines.

7

Chair Yoga for Building Strength

Does yoga really build muscle? Typically when people think of building muscle, they immediately think of weight lifting. However, you'd be surprised that yoga can help and support muscle gains, despite myths that may suggest otherwise. Likewise, you'd be surprised at how effective our body weight is for weight-loaded exercises. That said, the difference between a regular yoga flow and utilizing yoga for weight training is that you need to increase the number of sets and repetitions to boost muscle growth. You must also try changing your yoga variations occasionally while gradually increasing the difficulty. Like most things in life, when it becomes too easy, you need a new challenge to help you grow!

With each change you make in your yoga exercises, your muscles must learn how to manage the new tension they are under. In this case, take the poses you have learned throughout this book (plus the new ones we'll try in this chapter) and take them to the mat if you can. In other words, the chair is your foundation, and if you take a flow to a yoga mat, you now add a new challenge to the exercises and a new way to breathe life into your routine.

That sounds relatively straightforward, but one other component comes into play when building muscle: mechanical damage, which typically happens when we lift weights. Mechanical damage is when our muscle fibers are put under stress, which causes microscopic tears. (Tears are good unless you perform an exercise incorrectly.) When our muscles tear, they will heal and, as such, increase in size.

When we do yoga, mechanical damage will occur to our muscles in poses that we hold longer than usual. For example, if you do a reverse chair pose and hold it for a minute, your quadriceps muscles may begin to burn and feel fatigued. As a result, your leg muscles will tear microscopically and heal to build more muscle and increase their strength.

Metabolic stress, or "the burn," is another significant contributor to growing and sustaining muscle mass. For example, if you have ever done bicep curls and that last repetition felt like the hardest one of them all, you have put your muscles into metabolic stress because it feels like you cannot do that last rep (or others to come in subsequent sets). While you won't be doing bicep curls and sometimes trying to achieve metabolic stress while practicing yoga can be more complex unless you perform more challenging poses, so long as you apply resistance, mainly using your body weight, you can stimulate metabolic stress to force tension on your muscles. How much metabolic stress you put your muscles under depends on the variation and depth of your yoga poses. Don't worry; you don't need to worry about bulking up like Hulk Hogan. But remember, building strength is necessary to prevent falls, among other things. This chapter will look into different yoga routines that will help to increase your muscle strength.

Strength Building Routine 1

This is a great flow to build muscles in your legs. However, it's also an excellent routine to build core strength. Our core is at our center for a reason. It helps us perform almost every movement we need to do on a daily basis, such as getting out of bed or off the couch, walking up and down stairs, and bending over to pick things up.

We will dive into different exercises to help build your muscles, particularly your legs. We will be revisiting the following exercises:

- chair-supported downward dog (Chapter 4)
- seated bound angle pose (Chapter 4)
- seated eagle pose (Chapter 6)

Chair-Supported Boat Pose

Author John A. Shedd once said, "A ship in a harbor is safe, but that is not what ships are built for" (Shedd, 1928). It is a quote mistakenly attributed to Albert Einstein, which is beside the point. This is an important quote, as when you think about it, a ship leaving its harbor means the people steering it are leaving the comfort and protection of the harbor. As the boat pose is one of the more challenging poses to master, it can make us feel uncomfortable, just like a sailor setting out to sea.

From a yoga mythology perspective, it also has an interesting story! The waterways in India have a powerful symbolic signif- icance and are holy places in their culture. Many rivers throughout India are named after goddesses, such as Ganges, Sarasvati, and Yamuna.

In this story, Rama, his wife, Sita, and Rama's brother Lakshman were sent to exile from Ayodhya. On their journey to cross, they took the Ganges River, where they spotted a ferryman and called him over. Having known the story about Rama using the touch of his foot to turn a stone into a woman, the ferryman wondered if Rama would do the same with his boat.

Eventually, the ferryman agreed to carry the three across on the agreement that he could touch and wash Rama's feet. In Indian culture, it is a show of great respect, and it is believed that blessings are given when a revered person's foot is touched.

When the ferryman, Rama, Sita, and Lakshman arrived at their destination, the ferryman refused payment, acknowledging he and Rama were in the same profession where the ferryman carries people across a river but Rama carries them across the ocean of Samsara.

It's a beautiful story showing that the boat pose offers a lot of strength-building mechanics, both mentally and physically. You will initially notice how much your core muscles will burn because it activates all of your core muscles. Doing so will help you have better control over your range of motion and can improve back strength, specifically your lower back. Mentally, as you try to maintain the boat pose, you'll find it will enhance your focus and breathing. As there are a few ways to execute the boat pose, try each way to see which one will work best for you as a foundational point, and challenge yourself to make it harder when you get stronger.

Seated Boat Pose One Leg

In this first variation, you'll lift one leg and hold it in the position.

1. Begin by sitting in your chair in mountain pose with a tall spine. Your sit bones should be near the edge of the seat, but ensure your body feels stable and comfortable.
2. Lift your right leg and interlock your fingers behind your knee.
3. Engage your core as you hold the pose and avoid rounding your back.
4. Hold for about 30 seconds, then lower to switch legs.
5. Repeat three times with each leg lifted.

Helpful tip: Use a yoga block or a rolled-up pillow if you need additional support under your foot.

Seated Boat Pose One Leg and One Arm

You will lift your right leg with a bent knee and hold your right arm out for this variation, and ensure you do not round your back while holding the pose, and grab a yoga block or a rolled-up cushion if you need support under your foot on the floor.

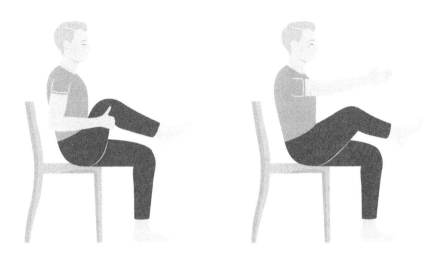

| Seated Boat Pose One Leg

Seated Boat Pose with Both Legs

In this variation, you will follow the same instructions as above, except this time, you will lift both legs and hold the back of your thighs with each hand.

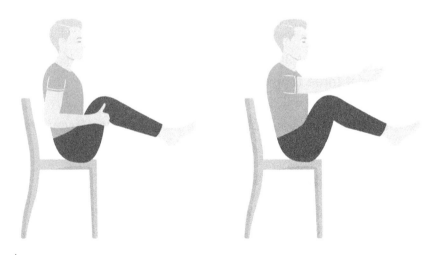

| Seated Boat Pose

Fully Seated Boat Pose

For the fully seated boat pose, you'll be holding your legs in the air and your arms forward. This is the most challenging way to execute the boat pose, so if you can't get it the first time, I know with practice and dedication, you'll get there!

Chair-Supported High Lunge

This high lunge with a chair will help support your leg so you can comfortably execute the pose. This pose is excellent for building strength in your hips, quadriceps, and calf muscles, which can help to improve your stability. It also helps to stretch your hip flexors which can become tight from too much sitting.

1. Begin by sitting in mountain pose on your chair.
2. Bring your right leg to the side of your chair as you turn your torso.
3. Using the chair for support, straighten your back leg with your toes curled under you. Rest your left hand on your leg.

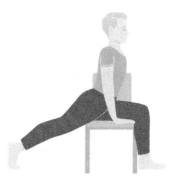

Chair-Supported Lunge Pose

4. As you hold the pose, ensure you engage your core muscles to find your balance.
5. If you feel stable, lift your arms above your head and hold.
6. When you are ready, lower your arms if you have them extended and bring your left leg in. Switch sides following the same steps.

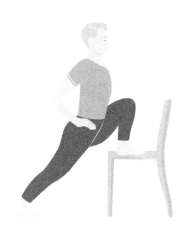

High Lunge Pose

For an added challenge, place your foot on the seat of the chair and your hands on your hips. This will really stretch and build muscle in your hip flexors.

Seated Camel Pose

Camels are fascinating creatures. When we picture them as animals, we likely imagine them helping people explore the great Egyptian pyramids. So what does a camel have to do with yoga?

Remember, yoga has many great lessons we can learn. While camels may be often associated with pyramids, it's good to remember that they can teach us great lessons, such as staying the course and trusting what will come.

The camel pose is a gentle backbend movement that will help improve your spine's flexibility while you open your chest and shoulders. As a result, you will find that your posture will get stronger when you implement the camel pose into your routine. In addition, you will want to use this pose in your strength-building routine to get more out of other strength-building exercises, in and outside of yoga.

1. Sit in your chair in mountain pose with your sit bones close to the front of the chair.
2. Roll your shoulders away from your ears and place your hands on your lower back with your elbows pointing behind you.

3. Gently lean your upper back to create a curve. If you can, lift your head to face the ceiling.
4. Take a few breaths before returning to the starting position. Repeat five times.

Putting Strength Building Routine 1 Together

To put this entire strength training routine together, here is what to do:

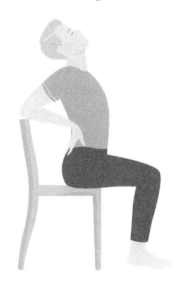

| Camel Pose

1. Begin by sitting tall on the edge of your chair with your feet flat on the floor. Roll your shoulders away from your ears and place your palms on your lower back, fingers pointing down and elbows pointing behind you. As you inhale, gently press your hips forward and arch your back, lifting your chest toward the ceiling. You should feel the stretch in your chest. After enjoying a few breaths in Camel Pose, return to a neutral seated position.
2. Move into the seated eagle pose by crossing your arms across your chest and touching the opposite shoulders with your right arm on top. Lift the back of your hands to meet each other in front of your face. If you want to go further, tuck your left hand so your fingers touch your right palm. Lift your elbows to deepen the stretch and remain here for a few breaths,

maintaining your posture. Slowly unwind your arms and let them rest in your lap.

3. You may also add your lower body to this exercise by crossing your right leg over your left and tucking your right foot behind your left calf.

4. From mountain pose, bring your right leg to the side of your chair as you turn your torso 90 degrees to the right. Place your palms on the chair's seat for support and straighten your back leg with your toes curled under you. Be sure to keep a tall spine and engage your core muscles to find your balance. If you are up for the challenge, lift your arms above your head, palms facing each other. After a few breaths, return to the center and repeat the exercise on your left side.

5. Slide to the front of your chair for the seated boat pose with one leg. Once you feel stable, lean back slightly, lift your right leg, and interlock your fingers behind your knee. Engage your core as you hold the pose and avoid rounding your back. Hold here for three long breaths before lowering your leg and switching sides. Aim to complete five repetitions.

6. After your last repetition, adjust yourself on your chair to ensure there's room for your feet to come together for the bound angle pose. Bring the soles of your feet together on your yoga block and let your knees drop to the sides. Hold for a couple of breaths.

7. Carefully return to a neutral seated position for the downward-facing dog pose. Stand up from your chair and turn so that you are facing the chair. Bend your torso toward the chair seat and take a couple of steps forward until your body forms a nice "V" shape, with your hips being the highest point. Press your palms

into the chair, draw your belly in, and push your hips back. Your head should be in line with your arms. On your last inhale, step toward your chair and slowly roll up to a standing position.

8. Repeat the flow two to three more times to build strength and endurance.

Strength Building Routine 2

This strength-building routine has similar benefits to the first strength routine but can be a little more challenging since it incorporates our ability to balance. So this flow can be a double whammy!

We will build strength with three new poses while implementing a few we've already done, including:

- reverse chair pose (Chapter 5)
- seated boat pose

Seated Twisted Chair

The twisted chair pose is another excellent pose for mobilizing your spine while strengthening your ankles, thighs, hip flexors, and glutes. I love this pose, especially because it challenges my balance and coordination.

1. Sit in your chair with your feet together. Squeeze your knees to activate your inner thigh muscles.
2. Bring your hands together in a prayer pose at the center of your chest.
3. As you hinge at your hips, twist your torso to the right so your elbow points to the ceiling. Place your left

elbow on the outside of your right knee.

4. Roll your right shoulder back and look up at the sky.
5. Hold for five breaths, then return to the starting position.
6. Switch sides.

When you build strength in this exercise, you should be able to lift your butt a few inches off of the seat.

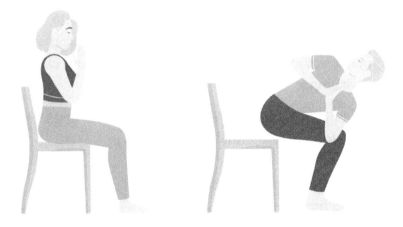

| Seated Twisted Chair Pose

Chair-Supported Upward Plank

The plank pose is an excellent full body exercise as it not only strengthens your core, but also your arms and shoulders. In a regular plank exercise, you face the floor. However, in the upward plank, your body will face upwards. Here's how to do it:

1. Begin in a seated mountain pose with your bottom close to the front of your chair seat.
2. Place your hands on either side of your bottom with your knuckles facing the front.

3. Extend your legs out in front of you on a diagonal with your toes flexed to the ceiling.
4. Press into your hands as you lift your bottom off of your chair to create a diagonal with your body. Ensure your core muscles are engaged.
5. Lower back down to your chair.

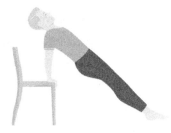

Modification: Planks are challenging for most of us! If you find extending your legs out in front of you difficult, keep your feet flat on the floor and bend your knees to 45 degrees. Engage your core and hold the plank.

Chair-Supported Upward Plank

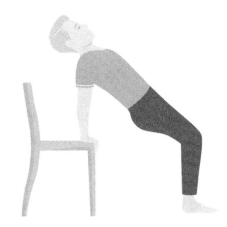

Modified Chair-Supported Upward Plank

Rag Doll

The rag doll pose is excellent for releasing tension in your legs, hips, and back to improve your overall flexibility.

1. Stand in front of your chair with your legs hip-distance apart.
2. Allowing your fingertips to lead the way, slowly roll forward as you bend at your hips.
3. Bring your arms together above your head, grabbing your elbows. Allow your head to hand between your arms.
4. Sway side to side in a gentle motion.
5. When you are ready, slowly roll back up.

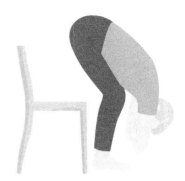

Ragdoll Pose

Helpful tip: If you find hanging freely difficult, rest your forearms on the chair seat.

Putting Strength Building Routine 2 Together

1. Let's start this strength training flow with the reverse chair pose. Slide to the edge of your chair, keeping your feet flat on the floor, hip-distance apart. On an inhale, lift your arms overhead with your palms facing each other, and fingers pointed to the ceiling. As you exhale, keep your spine straight and push your weight through your heels to stand up partially from your chair until your legs are at about 45 degrees. Hold here for about three to five breaths before slowly lowering back to your chair to return to a mountain pose to prepare for the seated boat pose.

2. Choose the boat pose variation you would like to complete. Once you feel stable, lean back slightly and lift one or both legs, interlocking your fingers behind the knee. Engage your core as you hold the pose and avoid rounding your back. If you're up for an added challenge, unlock your fingers and lift your arms out in front of you. Hold for three breaths before lowering one or both legs, returning to mountain pose.

3. Remaining seated toward the front of your chair, place your palms on the seat right behind your bottom with your knuckles facing the front for the upward plank pose. Extend both legs in front of you on a diagonal with your toes flexed to the ceiling. Pressing into your hands and engaging your core, lift your bottom off the chair to create a straight line with your body. Hold for two to three breaths before slowly lowering back down to your chair.

4. Reposition yourself back to mountain pose but with your feet together for the twisted chair pose. Squeeze your knees to activate your inner thigh muscles as you bring your hands to a prayer pose at the center of your chest. As you hinge at your hips, twist your torso to the right so your right elbow points to the ceiling and your left elbow rests outside your right knee. Be sure not to slouch your shoulders but to roll them back to create a straight line from elbow to elbow. Hold for five breaths before untwisting to return to the center.

5. To end the flow, stand up from your chair with your legs hip-distance apart. Allowing your fingertips to lead the way, slowly roll forward as you bend at the hips until you reach a comfortable position. Bend your arms above your head, grab your elbows, and allow

your head to hang between your arms. Gently sway side to side to help stretch your back and leg muscles. When you're ready, slowly roll back up.

6. Repeat all steps with the seated twisted chair pose going to the left.

Strength Building Routine 3

This flow is excellent for strengthening our quads, shoulders, arms, and core. This is one of the flows I use when looking for a quick full-body workout because the challenges built within it require a lot of control. In addition, it will combine multiple areas of focus into one.

We will use the following poses and a new one to boost strength in our legs and hips. These poses include:

- seated cat-cow from Chapter 3
- seated pigeon pose from Chapter 3
- seated yoga side bends from Chapter 3
- Warrior II from Chapter 4

Seated Extended Side Angle Pose

The seated extended side angle pose can help relieve stiffness in your shoulders, back, and side and build strength in your hips and quad muscles.

1. Begin in mountain pose.
2. Open your right leg to the outside of your chair, ensuring your knee is stacked over your ankle. Next, extend your left leg to the side with your toes pointed forward.

3. Rest your right forearm on your right leg as you extend your left arm above your head. If you can, turn your head to face your extended arm.
4. Come out of the pose by lowering your left arm and sitting back up. Repeat on the other side.

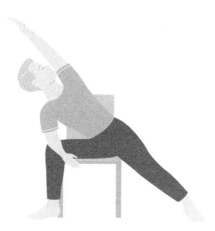

Seated Extended Side Angle Pose

Putting Strength Building Routine 3 Together

1. Start by sitting up tall toward the edge of your chair with your feet flat on the floor and your hands on your thighs. As you inhale, arch your back and push your chest out for the cow pose. As you exhale, round your back, pull your belly in, and let your head drop forward for the cat pose. Keep flowing between these two poses, syncing with your breath. From the cat pose, gently return to a neutral seated position for a seated side bend pose.
2. Inhale deeply as you raise your left arm overhead with your palm facing inward. Bring your right hand to the

side of the chair for stability—exhale as you bend toward your right, creating a "C" shape. You'll feel a nice stretch along your left side. From here, we will transition right into the extended side angle pose.

3. As you lean to your right, bring your right forearm down to rest on your right thigh and extend your left leg to the side with your toes pointing to the front. Hold for a few breaths before transitioning into Warrior I.

4. Keeping your legs and left arm still, engage your core as you raise your torso back to the center, rotate your shoulders to the right, and lift your right arm toward the sky. Your arms should be parallel with palms facing each other.

5. As you hold for three breaths, let's prepare to move into Warrior II. Rotate your shoulders to face the front and lower your arms to the side until they are at shoulder height. Hold here for three more breaths before lowering your arms, bringing your left leg to the center, and ending in mountain pose.

6. Wrapping up this strength-building flow is the seated pigeon pose. Place your left ankle over your right knee, creating a figure-four shape with your legs. If this feels good, you can stay here. If you want a deeper stretch, gently lean forward from your hips. You should feel a stretch in your right hip and bottom.

7. Repeat the flow two to three times, then switch sides to complete the flow two to three times on your left.

On top of building muscle, yoga can improve your flexibility as well. The next chapter will provide several chair yoga routines designed to enhance flexibility.

8
Chair Yoga for Flexibility

Did you know that by the time we get into our seventies, we lose up to 30% of our flexibility (Bataineh, n.d.)? This happens for many reasons, such as increased rigidity of the ligaments and tendons surrounding the joint, changes to the connective tissue collagen fibers that make up tendons and ligaments, and reduced elastin content that gives tendons and ligaments their elasticity. We also lose synovial fluid within the joint and a deterioration in the ligaments, cartilage, and tendons. It may seem like a lose-lose situation, especially when dealing with joint pain. Thankfully, dynamic stretching movements in chair yoga can help minimize discomfort.

The one thing you need to remember when experiencing joint pain is that remaining still causes more damage because you are not allowing the joint to find its range of motion (even if it's minimal). As the saying goes, if you don't use it, you'll lose it.

Yoga and chair yoga benefit people who have arthritis by getting movement back into their stiff joints. In general, stretching exercises help to increase and improve the range of motion in the joints. Since yoga and chair yoga encourage stretching throughout the practice, you get the best of both worlds: Pain and discomfort relief and an improved range of motion!

Flexibility Enhancing Routine 1

The beauty of this particular flow is that you can do it whenever your body feels ready for some gentle stretching. I personally find that incorporating it into your daily routine either in the morning or in the evening works like a charm.

We will revisit the following movements we have done in previous chapters:

- head and shoulder rolls (Chapter 6)
- seated cat-cow (Chapter 3)
- chair staff pose (Chapter 4).

Wrist Rolls

Aside from using our legs to walk, we use our hands and wrists for virtually everything we do, and it's often easy to take for granted until something, like a sore wrist, suddenly inhibits your ability to do something, like holding a grocery bag.

Our wrists make everything our hands do possible, so it is important to ensure they have an adequate range of motion to do simple activities without the nagging pain.

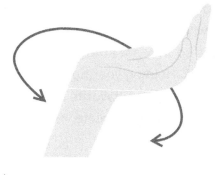

| Wrist Rolls

Wrist rolls are a simple exercise to execute and one you can do in and outside of your routine. Hold your hands slightly open, like holding a handful of chips you don't want to crush, and slowly circle your wrist 10 times clockwise. When you are done, go in the opposite direction. That's all there is to it! Super simple.

Putting Flexibility Enhancing Routine 1 Together

1. Start by sitting comfortably with your feet flat on the floor and your hands resting on your thighs or knees with a tall spine. Take a long, slow inhale. On the exhale, drop your chin to your chest and slowly roll your head clockwise in a big circle, letting it drop back, then to the right, forward, and left. Do this a few times in both directions. Be deliberate in your motions to ensure your neck is well cared for. Bring your head back up to a neutral position.

2. Lift your shoulders towards your ears, then roll them back, down, and forward in a circular motion. Start

with small rotations and gradually move into larger ones, then switch direction.

3. Lift your arms so they are straight in front of you to do some wrist rolls. Holding your hands slightly open (like holding a handful of your favorite snack), slowly rotate your wrists clockwise—complete 10 rotations before changing direction.

4. Place your hands on your thighs for the seated cat-cow pose. As you inhale, arch your back and roll your shoulders down, lifting your chest and gazing upwards for cow pose. As you exhale, round your spine, tuck your chin, and let your shoulders and head come forward for cat pose. Alternate between these two poses a few times, linking your breath with the movement. After your last round of cat-cow, take a moment to come back to a neutral spine.

5. Once you're sitting upright, extend your legs straight out in front of you, keeping your feet flexed and active. Place your hands behind your butt on the seat with your fingers facing the front and push into your hands to gently push your upper body forward until you feel a stretch in your calves and hamstrings. Return to the center to repeat the flow.

Flexibility Enhancing Routine 2

This particular yoga flow is perfect to kickstart your day or as a midday pick-me-up. It's like a burst of energy and relaxation combined! You can find a quiet and comfortable spot in your home where you can have some uninterrupted me-time. It could be your living room, bedroom, or even a peaceful corner in your backyard.

There are no new exercises in this second flexibility routine. It will include:

- shoulder rolls (Chapter 6)
- forward bend (Chapter 3)
- pigeon pose (Chapter 3)
- spinal twist (Chapter 3)
- seated goddess pose with a side bend (Chapter 5)
- seated camel pose (Chapter 7)

Putting Flexibility Enhancing Routine 2 Together

1. Let's begin this flexibility flow with shoulder rolls. Lift your shoulders towards your ears, then roll them back, down, and forward in a circular motion. Start with small rotations and gradually move into larger ones, then switch direction.
2. To move into the camel pose, roll your shoulders away from your ears and place your palms on your lower back, fingers pointing down and elbows pointing behind you. As you inhale, gently press your hips forward and arch your back, lifting your chest toward the ceiling. You should feel the stretch in your chest. After enjoying a few breaths in camel pose, return to a neutral seated position for a forward bend.
3. Take a big inhale and reach your arms towards the sky, lengthening your spine. As you exhale, fold forward from your hips, letting your hands rest on your shins, ankles, or the floor, depending on your flexibility. Let your head hang down for a few breaths,

feeling the gentle stretch in your back. When ready, roll your body back up to seated mountain pose.

4. From here, inhale and open your legs to a wide stance, turning your toes outward for the seated goddess pose. Raise your arms over your head with your palms facing each other and your fingers pointing to the sky. Then, bring your hands behind your head, interlocking your fingers. Exhale as you lean your torso sideways to the left, pointing your left elbow to the floor, feeling the stretch along your left side. After a few breaths, return to the center and bring your hands to your thighs.

5. Still focusing on stretching our right side, let's move into the pigeon pose. Place your right ankle over your left knee, creating a figure-four shape with your legs. Bring your hands to a prayer position and gently lean forward from your hips for an added stretch. You should feel a stretch in your right hip and bottom. After three breaths, lower your right foot to the floor and return to the center for a spinal twist.

6. To wrap up this flexibility flow, sit up tall, and as you exhale, twist your upper body to the right, placing your right hand on the back of the chair and your left hand on your right knee. Look over your right shoulder, hold for a few breaths, then inhale to return to the center.

7. Repeat the flow, focusing on your left side during steps four through six.

Flexibility Enhancing Routine 3

In this final flexibility routine, we will use wrist rolls, seated yoga side bends, seated cat-cow pose, and high-lunge with chair support to work on our flexibility, in addition to a new pose that will not only stretch our shoulders but also open our chest.

What I love most about the flexibility flows is that they aren't limited to a specific time and can be incorporated into various moments of your day. Whether during your morning routine, a midday break, or as part of your evening relaxation, find what works best for you and your schedule. As always, listen to your body and honor its needs. Your body may tell you when it is time to pause your day to focus on your flexibility.

Seated Cow Face

I admit, the name is a bit funny sounding. However, the pose got its name because your elbows look like cow's ears from the back.

Despite the hilarious name for this yoga pose, it has some awesome benefits, such as improving your posture, stretching your triceps, and working on shoulder mobility and flexibility. This is a great pose if you tend to sit more during the day to help counteract the slump many of us adopt when we sit. Here's how to do it:

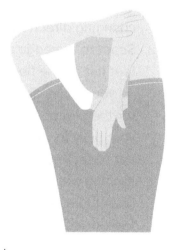

Seated Cow Face

1. Sit in your chair with your legs hip-distance apart.

2. Bring your right arm over your head and bend your elbow so your hand is along your spine with your fingers pointing down.
3. Use your left hand to bring your right elbow toward the left, allowing your right hand to slide down your spine.
4. Hold the pose for 30 seconds, then switch sides.

Putting Flexibility Enhancing Routine 3 Together

1. Let's start by warming up our bodies! Lift your arms so they are straight in front of you to do some wrist rolls. Holding your hands slightly open (like holding a handful of your favorite snack), slowly rotate your wrists clockwise—complete 10 rotations before changing direction.
2. Scoot to the edge of your chair with a tall spine, your feet flat on the floor, and your hands on your thighs. As you inhale, arch your back and push your chest out for the cow pose. As you exhale, round your back, pull your belly in, and let your head drop forward for the cat pose. Keep flowing between these two poses, syncing with your breath. From the cat pose, gently return to a neutral seated position for the seated cow-face stretch..
3. Bend your left arm at your elbow so your fingertips touch your shoulders. Reaching above your head with your right arm, grab your left elbow and gently pull to the right. Your left hand will shift down your spine as you get a nice shoulder, arm, and back stretch. After

three to five breaths, release your arm before switching sides to stretch your right shoulder.

4. After three to five breaths, inhale deeply as you release your right arm to raise overhead with your palm facing inward for the seated side bend. Bring your left hand to the side of the chair for stability— exhale as you bend toward your left, creating a "C" shape. You'll feel a nice stretch along your right side; hold for three breaths. From here, keep your left arm raised as you lift your torso back to a neutral position for the high lunge.

5. From mountain pose, bring your right leg to the side of your chair as you turn your torso 90 degrees to the right. Place your palms on the chair's seat for support and straighten your back leg with your toes curled under you. Be sure to keep a tall spine and engage your core muscles to find your balance. If you are up for the challenge, lift your arms above your head, palms facing each other. After a couple of breaths, return to center and repeat the exercise on your opposite side.

Though yoga is excellent for enhancing flexibility, it doesn't necessarily need to be about stretching. In fact, it can also be a great cardio workout. The next chapter will show you several different chair yoga routines that will get your blood pumping.

9
Chair Yoga for Cardio

When people think about doing yoga, it's common to associate the practice of it with one that will enhance flexibility and balance. We know this is true, but we must remember that yoga also boosts breathing exercises, meditation, and relaxation. In addition, these practices can enhance cardiovascular health by improving sleep patterns, reducing high blood pressure, and decreasing artery-damaging inflammation.

Hatha Yoga

Hatha yoga is a yoga practice done slowly using yoga postures and breath control. It focuses on breathing techniques as you hold one pose at a time to channel your energy source. There are many calming benefits to the practice from its slow pace, including:

- relieving symptoms of anxiety and depression

- relieving back pain
- improving balance
- promoting mindfulness
- enhancing mood and fatigue for people who have multiple sclerosis (MS)
- reducing neck pain
- improving stress management
- improving sleep

Hatha yoga may increase your heart rate, but not nearly as much as in a Vinyasa yoga practice.

Vinyasa Yoga

Vinyasa yoga is the opposite of Hatha yoga. Vinyasa focuses on stringing various poses together with synchronized breathing. As this yoga allows you to move continuously, you give your body a chance to increase its heart rate to have better circulation overall.

So, while people think that yoga is an activity you do to enhance flexibility and balance, it's clear that it can do much more! This chapter will go into flows you can use to improve cardiovascular health.

Chair Yoga Cardio Routine 1

Cardio is an important part of our health journey, so I try incorporating at least one cardio flow into my weekly routine. Since I'm still working full-time, I typically engage in this energizing cardio flow in the morning or before dinner. It's a great way to kickstart my day or boost my energy after a long day's work. Plus, I don't feel as guilty going back for a second helping at dinner.

In this first routine, we'll revisit the following exercises we have done in previous chapters to make up your flow:

- sun salutation (Chapter 3)
- seated pigeon pose (Chapter 3)
- Warrior II (Chapter 4)
- reverse Warrior pose (Chapter 4)
- seated goddess pose (Chapter 5)
- seated goddess pose with a twist (Chapter 5)
- extended side angle pose (Chapter 7)
- seated goddess pose forward fold (Chapter 7)

Putting Chair Yoga Cardio Routine 1 Together

It's time to get the heart pumping!

1. Let's start by sitting comfortably in your chair, feet planted firmly on the ground as we flow through the Seated Sun Salutation. Begin in a seated mountain pose with your knees stacked over your ankles, hip-distance apart. As you inhale deeply, lift your arms over your head, stretching them toward the sky. Exhale into a prayer pose as you bring your hands to your heart center. Keeping your hands in the same position, fold forward by hinging at your hips and rounding your spine. Release your hands, reaching them toward your feet. Inhale and roll up, imagining your vertebrae stacking on one another with your head lifting last. Lastly, roll your shoulders so they are

pulled away from your ears, and your hands rest on your thighs as you return to mountain pose.

2. For the pigeon pose, lift your right leg and cross your right ankle over your left knee. Bring your hands to a prayer position and gently lean forward from your hips for an added stretch. You should feel a stretch in your right hip and bottom. After three breaths, lower your right foot to the floor and move back to the center for Warrior II.

3. Shift to the right side of your chair, bring your right leg out to the side with your knee bent and your right foot flat on the floor. Extend your left leg behind you, toes pointing backward and resting on the floor. Extend your arms to the sides at shoulder height, your right arm pointing forward and your left arm pointing back, gazing over your right fingers. Hold for a few breaths before transitioning to reverse warrior.

4. Keeping your legs as they are, simply drop your left hand to rest on the back of your left leg and reach your right arm up towards the sky, creating a nice stretch on your right side. Remember to keep that right knee bent and hold your balance.

5. Holding the reverse warrior pose, let's transition to the seated extended side angle pose. Bring both arms back to shoulder height as you pass through Warrior II. Continue that motion and bring your right forearm down to rest on your right thigh while your left arm points to the sky. Turn your head to the left so you are gazing at your fingertips. Hold here for three breaths before bringing your torso and arms back to center, passing through warrior II again. As you keep moving,

bend your left leg and lift your arms for the goddess pose.

6. As you raise your arms over your head with your palms facing each other and your fingers pointing to the sky, adjust your feet by turning your toes outward and ensuring your knees remain stacked over your ankles. Then, bend your elbows to 90 degrees, palms facing forward, to create cactus arms.

7. Maintaining your goddess leg position, exhale as you twist your body to the right, grabbing the back of your chair with your right arm and resting your left hand on the outside of your right thigh. Hold here for a few breaths before you slowly untwist for a forward bend.

8. Move your hands to your inner thighs and inhale to engage your core muscles. As you exhale, hinge at your hips to fold your upper body forward, ensuring your neck and spine remain straight and connected. Reach for the floor, or rest your hands on your knees. Remember to listen to your body and only bend forward as far as what makes sense for you. Hang out here for a few breaths, releasing tension in your lower back and hips. Slowly lift your torso back up to the seated goddess pose.

9. Repeat this flow two or four times, ensuring you focus on the left and right sides.

Chair Yoga Cardio Routine 2

A vinyasa flow is not the only way to get cardio through yoga. You may want to incorporate a high-intensity interval training (HIIT) approach. Typically, HIIT is not recommended for seniors because it involves a lot of jumping. But, of course, we are doing everything through the comfort of a chair! To create the intensity you would be looking for, breathe in as you move into one and exhale for the next pose, repeating until your body feels fatigued.

This second cardio yoga routine I'm about to share with you is an energizing and invigorating sequence. It's best to practice it when you're looking for a boost of energy and want to get your blood flowing. In this routine, we will add a new exercise while revisiting the following exercises:

- seated twisted chair (Chapter 7)
- sun salutation (Chapter 3)
- seated-half wind relieving pose (Chapter 5)
- reverse chair (Chapter 5)
- seated boat pose (Chapter 7)

Seated Mountain Pose with Squats

This exercise is good for working on your coordination of getting out of a chair and back into it without support. Here is how to do the exercise:

1. Begin by sitting in your
2. chair with your hands hanging by your sides.
3. Extend your arms to shoulder height as you lift your bottom off of the chair into a standing position.
4. Slowly lower back down to your chair.
5. Stand back up and repeat steps two through four.

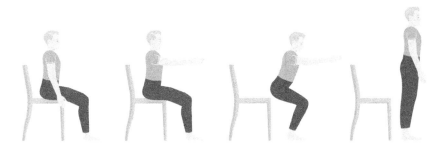

Seated Mountain Pose With Squats

Putting Chair Yoga Cardio Routine 2 Together

1. Let's get warmed up with the seated sun salutation! Begin in a seated mountain pose with your knees stacked over your ankles, hip-distance apart. As you inhale deeply, lift your arms over your head, stretching them toward the sky. Exhale into a prayer pose as you bring your hands to your heart center. Keeping your hands in the same position, fold forward by hinging at your hips and rounding your spine. Release your hands, reaching them toward your feet. Inhale and roll up, imagining your vertebrae stacking on one another with your head lifting last. Lastly, roll your shoulders so they are pulled away from your ears, and your hands rest on your thighs as you return to mountain pose to prepare for a twist.

2. Bring your feet together and squeeze your knees to activate your inner thigh muscles as you bring your hands to a prayer pose at the center of your chest. Twist your torso to the right so your right elbow points to the ceiling and your left elbow rests outside your right knee. Be sure not to slouch your shoulders but to

roll them back to create a straight line from elbow to elbow. Hold for three breaths before returning to the center. After three more breaths, return to the center and prepare to get those legs working. Extend your arms in front of you to shoulder height as you lift your bottom off the chair, just enough to engage your leg muscles but not enough to stand fully. Lower yourself back onto your chair, then stand up slightly again to repeat the process.

3. After your final squat, sit back on your chair to prepare for a bigger movement. Inhale deeply, and as you exhale, simultaneously press through your feet and raise your arms to shoulder height to stand up. Once standing, lower your arms back down to your sides. Inhale as you sit around down, your arms repeating the process. Repeat this a few times to sync your movement with your breath.

4. Now let's engage our core with the boat pose. With the desired pose variation in mind, lean back slightly and lift one or both legs, interlocking your fingers behind the knee. Engage your core as you hold the pose and avoid rounding your back. If you're up for an added challenge, unlock your fingers and lift your arms out in front of you. Hold for three breaths before lowering one or both legs, returning to mountain pose.

5. Repeat steps one through five before cooling down.

6. It's time to start cooling down with the camel pose. Place your palms on your lower back, fingers pointing down, and elbows pointing behind you. As you inhale, gently press your hips forward and arch your back, lifting your chest toward the ceiling. If you feel balanced, tilt your head back to gaze at the ceiling.

You should feel the stretch in your chest and core. After enjoying a few breaths in camel pose, return to a neutral seated position to wrap up this flow with the child's pose.

7. Open your legs to be slightly wider than hip-distance apart. Inhale to lengthen your spine, then exhale and fold forward, resting your arms on a chair seat in front of you or allowing your fingertips to reach the floor.

Chair Yoga Cardio Routine 3

I love this powerful cardio-focused yoga flow because it gets my heart pumping and energy soaring. When I'm ready to break a sweat, this is the flow I turn to. And remember, my yogi friends, the key to maximizing the benefits of this yoga flow is to move with intention, connect with your breath, and challenge yourself within your limits. Embrace the burn, but also listen to your body and make modifications as needed. Take breaks when necessary, and always prioritize your safety.

In this routine, we are revisiting:

- mountain pose with arms up (Chapter 3)
- chair-supported downward facing dog (Chapter 4)
- chair-supported upward plank (Chapter 7)
- chair-supported high lunge (Chapter 7)
- mountain pose with squats (Chapter 9)

Putting Chair Yoga Cardio Routine 3 Together

1. Let's start with mountain pose by sitting tall on the edge of your chair, feet flat on the floor, and hip-

distance apart. Inhale and reach your arms up overhead, bringing your palms together. For something a little different, lace your fingers together as you keep your index fingers and thumbs out to point to the ceiling. Exhale and roll your shoulders away from your ears. Hold here for five breaths before releasing your arms and slowly lowering them to the side until they reach the sides of your chair.

2. Place your palms on the seat right behind your bottom with your knuckles facing the front to prepare for the upward plank. Extend both legs in front of you on a diagonal with your toes flexed to the ceiling. Pressing into your hands and feet and engaging your core, lift your bottom off the chair to create a straight line with your body. Hold for two to three breaths before slowly lowering back to your chair and preparing to stand for mountain pose with squats.

3. From the seated mountain pose, inhale deeply, and as you exhale, simultaneously press through your feet and raise your arms to shoulder height to stand up. Once standing, lower your arms back down to your sides. Inhale as you sit back down, your arms repeating the process. Complete this pose a couple of times, and on your last repetition, remain standing.

4. Turn your body to face the seat of your chair. Take a step or two backward so you are a comfortable distance from the chair to do a high lunge. Place your left leg on the chair, pressing into both feet for support and placing your hands on your hips. Be sure to place your chair against a wall to avoid any unwanted movement. You can also turn the chair so that the chair back is on the side and hold onto it for

additional support. Hold the stretch for five breaths before switching sides.

5. Facing the chair seat, place your hands on the seat and walk your feet back until your body is in a straight line from head to heels. Engage your core and hold this plank for a few breaths.

6. To move from a plank to a downward-facing dog, engage your core to lift your hips and press them back to form the "V" shape. Maintaining your hands on the chair seat, press your chest toward your thigh. You should feel the stretch along your spine and the back of your legs. On your last inhale, step toward your chair and slowly roll up to a standing position.

You already know that yoga has numerous benefits, from strength training to working your heart. Well, it's only natural that it can also be an excellent tool for weight loss. The next chapter will provide several chair yoga routines for weight loss.

10
Chair Yoga for Weight Loss

Regularly practicing yoga and its benefits are extensive, from improving your flexibility, mobility, and balance to helping you improve your mental health. But does it really help you lose weight? It absolutely can help with weight management, so long as you pair it with a good diet filled with fruits, vegetables, whole grains, and healthy fats.

When you think about it, any physical activity can aid with weight loss and managing it. Yoga, especially more intense styles, is one of those other tools that can get your body moving in an enjoyable form, especially if walking is difficult for you on some days (or the weather is poor).

Additionally, people who are overweight or obese and practice yoga can see a decrease in their body mass index, according to the NCCIH (2020). Also, in comparing varying yoga programs for weight control supported by the NCCIH, the beneficial yoga programs were longer and more frequent and included:

- a dietary component to complement yoga practices.
- implementing other yoga elements.
- the ability to practice at home.

As yoga practices mindfulness on the mat, it gives you the skills to practice mindfulness off the mat too. In this case, mindfulness practice can lead you to mindful eating habits. For example, when we are hungry, we may overindulge to simmer the hunger craving. However, with mindful eating helping you understand a hunger cue, you can limit overeating. In addition, you may become more aware of what you are eating and begin to recognize what leaves you energized versus feeling bloated.

Stress is another contributing factor to weight gain. As yoga can help you manage your stress, your cortisol levels will have the chance to calm down thanks to the breathwork involved in yoga. Being highly stressed can make losing weight hard, especially if it triggers you to stress-eat and or you have trouble sleeping. However, as deep breathing can help reverse stress's adverse effects, it can make losing weight less stressful. (See what I did there?)

Yoga may involve slow, gentle movements, but because you are using your body weight, it gives your body a chance to build muscle. We discussed why building muscle through strength training is beneficial for various reasons, such as preventing you from falling, but it's also helpful in a weight loss regime.

What this should all tell you is that yoga is one of the ways that can help you live a healthier life. Holding too much weight has many health consequences. However, through yoga with other exercise routines, your body can start to lose weight.

Yoga Weight Loss Routine 1

Let's start with a power flow to support your weight loss goals. This sequence is all about building strength and kick-starting our metabolism. For maximum effectiveness, it's ideal to practice this yoga flow in the morning or early afternoon as it allows your body to wake up and energize for the day ahead fully.

In this first yoga weight loss routine, we will include a new exercise to help you build muscle and burn off fat for weight loss. In addition, we will be resuming the following exercises:

- chair-supported downward facing dog (Chapter 4)
- chair-supported upward facing dog (Chapter 4)
- triangle pose (Chapter 4)
- chair-supported high lunge (Chapter 7)

Standing Wind-Relieving Pose

The standing wind-relieving pose is the standing variation to the seated version from Chapter 5. You should find that you will get a deeper stretch in your glutes when you pull your leg into your chest. Here's how to do it:

1. Stand with the back of your chair facing your left side. Place your left hand on the backrest for support with your right hand on your hip.
2. Bring your right leg up as high as it can go. You have the option to grab your knee with your right hand to

bring it closer to your chest. Ensure that your spine remains straight.

3. Hold for a few moments, then lower back down. Complete 10 repetitions before switching sides.

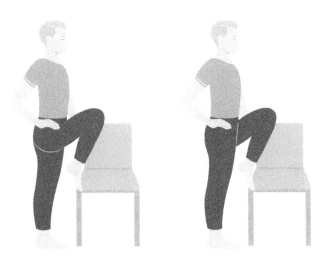

| Standing Wind-Relieving Pose

Putting Yoga Weight Loss Routine 1 Together

1. Let's begin with the downward-facing dog pose. Standing a little distance from the front of the chair, bend your torso toward the chair's seat and adjust your feet until your body forms a nice "V" shape, with your hips being the highest point. Press your palms into the chair, draw your belly in, and push your hips back. Your head should be in line with your arms. Hold here for a couple of breaths.

2. We will first pass through the chair-supported plank pose to move into the upward-facing dog pose. Hinging at the hips, shift your weight forward until

your body is straight from head to heels. Engage your core as you hold here for a few breaths.

3. After your last exhale, inhale and lift your chest until you have a slight bend in your back, then exhale to deepen the backbend to your comfort level. Hold for two more breaths. Walk your feet toward the front of the chair until you reach a standing position.

4. Moving into the triangle pose, step your right foot forward so it's just behind the chair and your left foot back about two to three steps with toes facing the front. Shift your left hip back and bring your right hand down until it reaches the chair seat while you extend your left arm toward the ceiling. Turn your head to the left to gaze up toward your fingertips. This should create a nice straight line from your left hand to your right. Remember to keep both legs straight and your chest open as you hold for three breaths.

5. Step to the side of your chair so that the back is on your left side for the standing wind-relieving pose. Place your left hand on the backrest and your right hand on your hip. Ensure your spine remains straight, and lift your right leg as high as possible. If you'd like, you can use your right hand to bring your leg closer to your chest. Hold this pose briefly before lowering your leg and preparing for a high lunge.

6. Turn the chair to place your left hand on the backrest and your right foot on the chair seat. Adjust your feet until you are comfortable from the chair to make a high lunge. Place your right leg on the chair, pressing into both feet for support and placing your hands on your hips. Hold the stretch for five breaths before returning your foot to the floor.

7. Repeat all the steps, focusing on your left side for the standing wind-relieving pose and the high lunge with chair support.

Yoga Weight Loss Routine 2

When I need a pick-me-up, I love turning to this flow. Not only does it help me burn calories, but I usually finish the flow feeling accomplished and awesome about myself! The key to maximizing the weight loss benefits of this yoga flow is to move mindfully, connect with your breath, and challenge yourself within your limits.

In this second routine, we will revisit the following exercises:

- Warrior II pose (Chapter 4)
- reverse Warrior pose (Chapter 4)
- reverse chair pose (Chapter 5)
- seated boat pose (Chapter 7)
- seated extended side angle pose (Chapter 7)

Putting Yoga Weight Loss Routine 2 Together

1. Begin in a seated mountain pose with your hands on your knees. On an inhale, lift your arms overhead with your palms facing each other, and fingers pointed to the ceiling. As you exhale, keep your spine straight and push your weight through your heels to stand up partially from your chair until your legs are at about 45 degrees. Hold here for about three to five breaths before shifting to sit squarely on your chair again, preparing for the seated boat pose.

2. With the desired pose variation in mind, slide to the front of the chair, lean back slightly, and lift one or both legs, interlocking your fingers behind the knee. Engage your core as you hold the pose and avoid rounding your back. If you're up for an added challenge, unlock your fingers and lift your arms out in front of you. Hold for three breaths before lowering one or both legs, returning to mountain pose for warrior II.

3. Shift to the right side of your chair, extending your right leg out to the side with your knee bent and your right foot flat on the floor. Extend your left leg behind you, toes pointing backward and resting on the floor. Extend your arms to the sides at shoulder height, your right arm pointing forward and your left arm pointing back, gazing over your right fingers. Hold for a few breaths before transitioning to reverse warrior.

4. Keeping your legs as they are, simply drop your left hand to rest on the back of your left leg and reach your right arm up towards the sky, creating a nice stretch on your right side. Remember to keep that right knee bent and hold your balance.

5. Holding the reverse warrior pose, let's transition to the seated extended side angle pose. Bring both arms to shoulder height as you pass back through Warrior II. Continue that motion and bring your right forearm down to rest on your right thigh while your left arm points to the sky. Turn your head to the left so you are gazing at your fingertips. Hold here for three breaths before repeating the routine.

Yoga Weight Loss Routine 3

To enhance our weight loss journey, this flow pulls double duty and also works on cardio. This is a great flow to help us increase our endurance, benefiting us even more in the long run. I love starting my day with this flow because it kick starts metabolism and gives our body a wake-up call. Not to mention it helps us burn those calories!

In this final routine, we will revisit the following exercises:

- Warrior I and II poses (Chapter 4)
- reverse Warrior pose (Chapter 4)
- seated twisted chair pose (Chapter 7)
- chair-supported downward dog pose (Chapter 4)
- triangle pose (Chapter 4)

Putting Yoga Weight Loss Routine 3 Together

For this flow, it is important that your chair is on a yoga mat or placed against a wall to avoid any unwanted movement.

1. Let's kick off this routine with the triangle pose. Start by standing in front of your chair with your feet hip-distance apart. Step your right foot forward so it's just behind the chair and your left foot back about two to three steps with toes facing the front. Shift your left hip back and bring your right hand down until it reaches the chair seat while you extend your left arm toward the ceiling. Turn your head to the left to gaze up toward your fingertips. This should create a nice straight line from your left hand to your right.

Remember to keep both legs straight and your chest open as you hold for three breaths.

2. Moving into a downward-facing dog, rotate your shoulders to the right until they are facing the chair seat. Place your hands on the seat shoulder-width apart before adjusting your feet to form the iconic 'V' shape. Press your palms into the chair, draw your belly in, and push your hips back. Your head should be in line with your arms. Hold here for a few breaths before walking your feet back toward the chair for Warrior I.

3. Take a seat on the edge of your chair, sit up nice and tall with your feet flat on the ground. Rotate to the right so your right leg is bent over the side of the chair and your right foot is flat on the floor. Extend your left leg behind you, toes pointed back, and resting on the ground. Sweep your arms up towards the sky and take a moment to find your balance.

4. While maintaining your leg positions, simply rotate your upper body to the left, lowering your arms to the sides at shoulder height, your right arm pointing forward, and your left arm pointing back.

5. Keeping your legs as they are, drop your left arm down to rest on the back of your left leg and reach your right arm up towards the sky, creating a nice stretch on your right side. Remember to keep that right knee bent and hold your balance. After three breaths, slowly lift your torso and bring your body back to the center.

6. Reposition yourself back to mountain pose but with your feet together for the twisted chair pose. Squeeze your knees to activate your inner thigh muscles as you bring your hands to a prayer pose at the center of your chest. As you hinge at your hips, twist your torso to

the right so your right elbow points to the ceiling and your left elbow rests outside your right knee. Be sure not to slouch your shoulders but to roll them back to create a straight line from elbow to elbow. Hold for five breaths before untwisting to return to the center.

7. Repeat the flow, focusing on the left side.

There you have it! A complete collection of chair yoga routines that are perfect for getting you started on your yoga journey.

Beyond The Pages

Are you ready to spread good vibes and help others on their wellness journey?

Let me ask you this: Have you ever experienced the joy of being part of something bigger than yourself? That feeling of fulfillment when you know you've made a positive difference in someone's life? Well, get ready because here's your chance to be a superhero for seniors!

Chair Yoga for Seniors has the power to make a big difference. This little treasure is packed with wisdom and tailored specifically for our beloved seniors who deserve to live their lives to the fullest. But here's the exciting part – your review can impact countless others too!

Leaving an honest review for *Chair Yoga for Seniors* is an opportunity to deliver value to many individuals seeking a healthier and happier lifestyle. Your feedback can guide them toward pain relief, fall prevention, and increased mobility. By sharing your experience, you'll be helping those looking for effective ways to overcome physical challenges and reclaim their independence.

Now, let's cut to the chase: I'm here to ask you, with all my yogic heart, to take a moment and leave an honest review for *Chair Yoga for Seniors: Relieve Pain, Prevent Falls, and Boost Mobility for Greater Independence*. Your review can work wonders! Head to Amazon and click that magical "Leave a Review" button. It's time to spread the love!

By leaving a review, you're not only helping potential readers make an informed decision, but you're also contributing to a positive ripple effect in the lives of others. Your words can uplift spirits, ignite motivation, and pave the way for newfound self-care journeys. Plus, your review supports the amazing author who poured their heart and soul into creating this gem, helping them reach even more individuals in need.

But here's an added bonus: Your kindness won't go unnoticed! By leaving a review, you become part of a community of kind-hearted souls who inspire and uplift one another.

Entrepreneurs and authors thrive on positive feedback, and your support may lead to exciting collaborations and opportunities in the future. Good karma is never wasted!

So, my fellow yogis, let's join forces and create a wave of positivity. Leave an honest review for *Chair Yoga for Seniors*, and let's empower countless individuals to embark on their own transformative wellness journeys. Together, we can make a lasting impact and help others find the strength, balance, and joy they deserve.

Thank you for being an incredible part of this compassionate community. Your review matters, and I can't wait to see the amazing impact we'll create together!

Namaste, and keep shining your light!

P.S. Remember to share specific details about how the book resonated with you, any breakthroughs you experienced, and how it brought positivity into your life. Your unique perspective will make your review truly remarkable!

Using your phone's camera, scan the code below to leave a review on Amazon.com.

With gratitude and grace,

~Jackie

Conclusion

Yoga is one of the best and most gentle exercises you can do for yourself and your aging body. Yoga, whether on the mat or done from a chair, gives our body a chance to breathe in new ways, and that isn't just on the mindfulness side of things.

Chair yoga is a seamless way for you to practice this ancient art in a supported manner, especially when some yoga postures are complex. It's excellent for seniors with an issue with their range of motion due to arthritis and difficulty balancing or moving their body for any other reason.

Yoga's mindfulness allows you to be fully aware of how your body feels through each pose, including the sequence that connects one pose to the next. Chair yoga will enable seniors to enhance their overall physical well-being regardless of their fitness level. Chair yoga allows for better flexibility so your joints can move through their range of motion, improve your strength and bone health so you can balance better, improve your posture, and manage your pain. In addition, yoga can help you manage your weight and mental well-being and boost your energy so you can do what you love throughout the day and sleep well at night. Thus being mindful certainly can do a lot for us!

Being on a chair versus a mat for yoga can feel strange, especially if you are a seasoned yogi. But never fear whether your yoga routine will suffer. Yes, some poses will feel awkward at first, but if you go into your session thinking about only that, it will impact how much your yoga session will not be as beneficial as you want it to be. That said, ensure you set a goal for yourself and understand the intentions to get to your goal. Without the steps (intentions), you will lack the motivation to keep up with your yoga routine. So, for example, if you want to practice chair yoga to reduce and manage pain associated with arthritis, understand what is happening now with your body and what you need to do to help manage your pain. Maybe it's first focusing on flexibility in a specific area to reclaim mobility. Whatever it is, make it purposeful. Be kind if your body is moving slowly today, and notice if your thoughts wander off so you can bring them back into your present focus.

In this book, we have looked at various techniques and flows that you can incorporate into 5 to 10 minutes of your day. These flows included:

- **Warming up:** Warming up allows your body to increase blood flow to your muscles to prepare for the upcoming yoga poses.
- **Cooling down:** Cooling down after your yoga session allows your body to take in all the benefits you gained

from your practice. Plus, it allows your body to slow down instead of stopping suddenly.

- **Balance focus:** As falling is one of the leading reasons seniors end up hospitalized, maintaining balance is critical for your physical well-being. You now have three different chair yoga flows you can utilize to focus on your balance so you can be prepared for anything that wants to knock you down.
- **Easing joint and arthritic pain:** As chair yoga is low impact, your joints will thank you because you can use this exercise method to work through the pain in a gentle motion.
- **Strength building:** Yoga from a chair, at first glance, may not seem like you can increase your strength, but with some challenging flows, you can build muscle which helps with various things, such as minimizing fall risks.
- **Increasing flexibility:** We discussed how chair yoga is therapeutic for aches and pains due to arthritis or other reasons. However, maintaining flexibility is critical to keeping your independence because it prevents you from losing your range of motion.
- **Cardio:** Yoga and cardio may seem to make a strange mix, but you would be surprised by how much your heart rate can increase your cardiovascular health when you take your practice up a notch!
- **Weight loss:** Any exercise is beneficial for maintaining your weight or for a weight loss program. When paired with eating well, yoga can help you lose weight by using your body weight. However, the mindful practices in yoga will also train your brain to

be aware of your eating and recognize hunger
triggers.

Yoga, whether you are seasoned or not, has its challenges. For example, Jane went from being a non-yogi to someone who tries to practice at least three times a week because it keeps her body flexible and ready for her other activities!

Now that you have started with these easy chair yoga routines, it's time to develop your yoga skills further. So keep going with yoga and continue to experience its benefits! If you are looking for other ways to incorporate fitness into your life, check out my other books in this series.

Always a sign of gratitude to you and your practice,

~Jackie

Also by Jackie Jacobs

Fitness Freedom for Seniors: 20 Simple Yoga Positions to Regain Your Strength and Independence

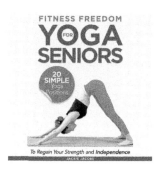

Fitness Freedom for Seniors: 15-Minute Strength Training Workouts to Reclaim Your Balance, Energy, and Confidence

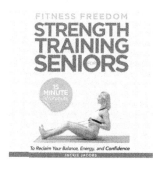

Bibliography

admin. (2020, May 3). *10 seated yoga poses for seniors.* Yoga Poses Basic. https://yogaposesbasic.com/seated-yoga-poses-for-seniors/

American Heart Association editorial staff. (2014, September 1). *Warm up, cool down.* American Heart Association. https://www.heart.org/en/healthy-living/fitness/fitness-basics/warm-up-cool-down

Arthritis. (2021, April 15). Cleveland Clinic. https://my.clevelandclinic.org/health/diseases/12061-arthritis

Baiera, V. (2021, June 15). *The benefits of chair Yoga for seniors.* Step2Health. https://step2health.com/blogs/news/benefits-of-chair-yoga-for-seniors

Bataineh, A. (n.d.). *Why we lose flexibility with age and what to do about it.* Span. https://www.span.health/blog/why-we-lose-flexibility-with-age-and-what-to-do-about-it

Beisecker, L. (2021, August 2). *The Holistic Benefits of Cat/Cow Pose.* DoYou. https://www.doyou.com/the-holistic-benefits-of-catcow-pose-56731

Benefits of bringing a friend to yoga class. (2021, October 15). Asheville Yoga Center. https://www.youryoga.com/benefits-of-bringing-a-friend-to-yoga-class/

Berstein, S. (n.d.). *Yoga benefits for arthritis.* Arthritis Foundation. https://www.arthritis.org/health-wellness/healthy-living/physical-activity/yoga/yoga-benefits-for-arthritis

Bestor, S. M. (n.d.). *10 tips to get the most out of your yoga class.* Yoga International. https://yogainternational.com/article/view/10-tips-to-get-the-most-out-of-your-yoga-class/

Bilski, R. (2018, December 21). *Why we twist in yoga: the benefits of this simple action.* Yogapedia. https://www.yogapedia.com/why-we-twist-in-yoga-the-benefits-of-this-simple-action/2/11287

Blaszczak, J. (2016, May 17). *Get in the Right Mindset to Exercise Regularly.* Psych Central. https://psychcentral.com/lib/get-in-the-right-mindset-to-exercise-regularly

Buckner Parkway Place. (2022, November 5). *5 Benefits of Chair Yoga for Seniors.* https://bucknerparkwayplace.org/news-blog/5-benefits-of-chair-yoga-for-seniors/

Campbell, B. (2020, May). *Bone health basics.* OrthoInfo. https://orthoinfo.aaos.org/en/staying-healthy/bone-health-basics

Carter, A. (n.d.). *10 health benefits of child's pose.* Yoga Practice. https://yo-gapractice.com/yoga/10-health-benefits-of-childs-pose/

Chai, C. (2023, May 7). *Can Yoga Help You Lose Weight?* EverydayHealth. https://www.everydayhealth.com/yoga/big-ways-yoga-can-help-with-your-weight-loss-goals/

Chair wide legged seated twist yoga. (n.d.). Tummee.com. https://www.tummee.com/yoga-poses/chair-wide-legged-seated-twist

CNY Healing Arts. (2010, October 15). *The health benefits of Baddha Konasana (Bound Angle Pose).* https://www.cnyhealingarts.com/the-health-benefits-of-baddha-konasana-bound-angle-pose/

Contie, V. (2011, October 31). *Yoga or stretching eases low back pain.* National Institutes of Health. https://www.nih.gov/news-events/nih-research-matters/yoga-or-stretching-eases-low-back-pain

Cronkleton, E. (2019, October 23). *Boost your yoga flexibility with these 8 yoga poses* (J. Keiter, Ed.). Healthline. https://www.healthline.com/health/exercise-fitness/yoga-for-flexibility#shoulder-flexibility

Cronkleton, E. (2021, August 11). *Yoga for weight loss* (S. Ullman, Ed.). Healthline. https://www.healthline.com/health/yoga-for-weight-loss

Davidson, K. (2021, May 4). *Pigeon pose: a how-to guide* (S. Ward, Ed.). Health-line. https://www.healthline.com/health/fitness/pigeon-pose

DeCataldo, J. (2023, January 1). *Chair yoga and why seated yoga poses are good for you.* Lifespan. https://www.lifespan.org/lifespan-living/chair-yoga-and-why-seated-yoga-poses-are-good-you

Dellwo, A. (2022, July 4). *The benefits of yoga for people with fibromyalgia.* Verywell Health. https://www.verywellhealth.com/yoga-for-fibromyalgia-715782

Derrick. (n.d.). *Chair yoga for Seniors - 17 great stretches.* ElderGURU. https://www.elderguru.com/chair-yoga-for-seniors-17-great-stretches/

Exercise 101: don't skip the warm-up or cool-down. (2020, July 20). Harvard Health Publishing; Harvard Health Medical School. https://www.health.harvard.edu/staying-healthy/exercise-101-dont-skip-the-warm-up-or-cool-down

Ezrin, S. (2021, December 14). *16 benefits of yoga that are supported by science* (S. Ward, Ed.). Healthline. https://www.healthline.com/nutrition/13-benefits-of-yoga

Falkenberg, R. I., Eising, C., & Peters, M. L. (2018). Yoga and immune system functioning: a systematic review of randomized controlled trials. *Journal of Behavioral Medicine, 41*(4), 467–482. https://doi.org/10.1007/s10865-018-9914-y

5 Chair Exercises That Reduce Belly Fat In No Time! (n.d.). *David Wolfe. https://www.davidwolfe.com/5-chair-exercises-reduce-belly-fat/*

Goddess pose hands behind head side bend yoga. (n.d.). Tummee.com. https://www.tummee.com/yoga-poses/goddess-pose-hands-behind-head-side-bend

Goddess pose hands knees forward bend pose. (n.d.). Tummee.com. https://www.tummee.com/yoga-poses/goddess-pose-hands-knees-forward-bend-pose-chair/benefits

Goddess pose on chair. (n.d.). Tummee.com. https://www.tummee.com/yoga-poses/goddess-pose-on-chair

Houlis, A. (2021, December 16). *Learn How to Set Intentions Correctly for the Biggest Impact.* Shape. https://www.shape.com/lifestyle/mind-and-body/mental-health/how-to-set-intentions

How much physical activity do older adults need? (2023, April 13). Centers for Disease Control and Prevention. https://www.cdc.gov/physicalactivity/basics/older_adults/index.htm

How to do seated hip circles chair. (n.d.). Tummee.com. https://www.tummee.com/yoga-poses/seated-hip-circles-chair/how-to-do

How to get started with chair yoga. (n.d.). University of Arkansas System. https://www.uaex.uada.edu/life-skills-wellness/health/physical-activity-resources/chair-yoga.aspx

How yoga may enhance heart health. (2019, April 1). Harvard Health Publishing; Harvard Medical School. https://www.health.harvard.edu/heart-health/how-yoga-may-enhance-heart-health

Hoy, D., March, L., Brooks, P., Blyth, F., Woolf, A., Bain, C., Williams, G., Smith, E., Vos, T., Barendregt, J., Murray, C., Burstein, R., & Buchbinder, R. (2014). The global burden of low back pain: estimates from the Global Burden of Disease 2010 study. *Annals of the Rheumatic Diseases, 73*(6), 968–974. https://ard.bmj.com/content/73/6/968.long

Khayela, A. (2022, September 2). *Does yoga build muscle?* LiveScience. https://www.livescience.com/does-yoga-build-muscle#section-progressive-overload-through-pose-progression

Kovar, E. (2015, June 18). *Chair yoga poses | 7 poses for better balance.* American Council on Exercise. https://www.acefitness.org/resources/everyone/blog/5478/chair-yoga-poses-7-poses-for-better-balance/

Lewis, A. (2021, November 8). *Sun Salutations Explained—and why you should master them.* Byrdie. https://www.byrdie.com/sun-salutation

Lindberg, S. (2021, November 5). *These Yoga Moves Can Be Part of a Great Cardio Workout.* SheKnows. https://www.sheknows.com/health-and-wellness/articles/1836563/yoga-cardio-workout/

MasterClass. (n.d.). *Chair pose in yoga: 5 benefits of Utkatasana.* https://www.masterclass.com/articles/awkward-chair-pose

Matthews, J. (2013, June 21). *How to get more out of your yoga practice*. American Council on Exercise. https://www.acefitness.org/resources/everyone/blog/3383/how-to-get-more-out-of-your-yoga-practice/

Mayo Clinic Staff. (2021, October 6). *Aerobic exercise: how to warm up and cool down*. Mayo Clinic. https://www.mayoclinic.org/healthy-lifestyle/fitness/in-depth/exercise/art-20045517

Mayo Clinic Staff. (2022, April 28). *Relaxation techniques: try these steps to reduce stress*. Mayo Clinic. https://www.mayoclinic.org/healthy-lifestyle/stress-management/in-depth/relaxation-technique/art-20045368

McGee, K. (2017, February 27). *Chair yoga warm-ups: poses to get your blood flowing*. Kristin McGee. https://kristinmcgee.com/chair-yoga-warm-ups

Merriam-Webster. (n.d.-a). *Goal*. https://www.merriam-webster.com/dictionary/goal

Merriam-Webster. (n.d.-b). *Intention*. https://www.merriam-webster.com/dictionary/intention

Navasana (boat pose). (2020, May 27). Flex Hot Yoga. https://flexhotyoga.com.au/blog/pom-navasana

NCCH Clinical Digest for Health Professionals. (2020, February). *Yoga for health: what the science says*. National Center for Complementary Integrative Health. https://www.nccih.nih.gov/health/providers/digest/yoga-for-health-science#:~:text=National%20survey%20data%20show%20that%206.7%20percent%20of

Neubauer, D. N. (1999). Sleep Problems in the Elderly. *American Family Physician*, 59(9), 2551–2558. https://www.aafp.org/pubs/afp/issues/1999/0501/p2551.html

9 benefits of yoga. (n.d.). Johns Hopkins Medicine. https://www.hopkinsmedicine.org/health/wellness-and-prevention/9-benefits-of-yoga

Noel, S. (2022, November 29). *Bound Angle pose*. Lessons. https://lessons.com/yoga-poses/bound-angle-pose

Pizer, A. (2020, September 15). *How to do reverse Warrior (Viparita Virabhadrasana) in yoga*. Verywell Fit. https://www.verywellfit.com/reverse-Warrior-pose-3567108

Pizer, A. (2021a, August 9). *Basic and advanced seated yoga poses*. Verywell Fit. https://www.verywellfit.com/seated-yoga-poses-3567037

Pizer, A. (2021b, December 8). *How to do cat-cow stretch (Chakravakasana) in yoga*. Verywell Fit. https://www.verywellfit.com/cat-cow-stretch-chakravakasana-3567178

Pizer, A. (2022a, August 22). *Introduction to vinyasa flow yoga*. Verywell Fit. https://www.verywellfit.com/introduction-to-vinyasa-flow-yoga-4143120

Pizer, A. (2022b, November 4). *10 yoga poses you can do in a chair*. Verywell Fit. https://www.verywellfit.com/chair-yoga-poses-3567189

Pizer, A. (2022c, November 4). *What to expect from a hatha yoga class*. Verywell Fit. https://www.verywellfit.com/what-is-hatha-yoga-3566884

Posture of the month: Navasana (boat pose). (2020, May 27). Flex Hot Yoga. https://flexhotyoga.com.au/blog/pom-navasana

Ragdoll pose. (n.d.). Yogapedia. https://www.yogapedia.com/definition/10505/ragdoll-pose#:~:text=Releases%20tension%20in%20the%20lower

Reid-St. John, S. (2013, March 12). *Top chair yoga poses for strength*. Spry Living. https://spryliving.com/articles/top-chair-yoga-poses-for-strength/

Revolved chair pose. (n.d.). YogaClassPlan.com. https://www.yogaclassplan.com/yoga-pose/revolved-chair-pose/

Romine, S. (2023, March 3). *43 yoga quotes to inspire your practice*. BODi. https://www.beachbodyondemand.com/blog/inspirational-yoga-quotes

Saal, K. (2019, February 19). *What is Vinyasa Yoga?* One Flow Yoga. https://oneflowyoga.com/blog/what-is-vinyasa-yoga

Sankhe, A. (2022, November 16). *Benefits of Garudasana (eagle pose) and how to do it by Dr. Ankit Sankhe*. PharmEasy. https://pharmeasy.in/blog/health-fitness-benefits-of-garudasana-and-how-to-do-it/

Sassos, S. (2023, January 4). *Is Yoga an Effective Way to Lose Weight?* Good Housekeeping. https://www.goodhousekeeping.com/health/fitness/a42216562/yoga-for-weight-loss/

Sawruk, C. (2019, December 12). *Why setting intentions is the way to achieve your goals*. Medium. https://coraliesawruk.medium.com/why-setting-intentions-is-the-way-to-achieve-your-goals-76d5e026d5d5#:~:text=Setting%20intentions%20is%20the%20act

Shedd, J. A. (1928). *Salt from my attic*. Mosher Press.

Side bending poses. (n.d.). YogaBasics. https://www.yogabasics.com/practice/pose-type/side-bending-poses/

Six relaxation techniques to reduce stress. (2022, February 2). Harvard Health Publishing; Harvard Health Medical School. https://www.health.harvard.edu/mind-and-mood/six-relaxation-techniques-to-reduce-stress

Stelter, G. (2020, May 29). *7 yoga poses you can do in a chair*. Healthline. https://www.healthline.com/health/fitness-exercise/chair-yoga-for-seniors

Styx, L. (2021, October 19). *Why We Set Intentions in Yoga and Meditation Practice*. Verywell Mind. https://www.verywellmind.com/why-we-set-intentions-in-yoga-and-meditation-practice-5205511

Sullivan, C. (2021, June 24). *The benefits of standing tall in Tadasana (mountain pose)* (A. DeLucca, Ed.). Healthline. https://www.healthline.com/health/fitness-exercise/tadasana-benefits

Toli, A., Webb, T. L., & Hardy, G. E. (2015). Does forming implementation intentions help people with mental health problems to achieve goals? A meta-analysis of experimental studies with clinical and analogue samples. *British Journal of Clinical Psychology, 55*(1), 69–90. https://doi.org/10.1111/bjc.12086

Try these yoga poses to improve your flexibility. (2022, September 26). Cleveland Clinic. https://health.clevelandclinic.org/yoga-poses-improve-flexibility/

12 simple and easy yoga for hip pain poses to find relief. (n.d.). Pain Doctor. https://paindoctor.com/yoga-for-hip-pain/

Ulu Contributor. (2023, April 4). *How to do chair yoga poses: a guide to getting started.* Ulu Yoga. https://www.uluyoga.com/how-to-do-chair-yoga-poses-a-guide-to-getting-started/

Upward Facing Dog pose. (n.d.). Raj Yoga. https://rajyogarishikesh.com/upward-facing-dog-pose.html

Upward Facing Dog Pose with chair steps. (n.d.). Tummee.com. https://www.tummee.com/yoga-poses/upward-facing-dog-pose-with-chair/steps

Upward plank pose hands chair. (n.d.). Tummee.com. *https://www.tummee.com/yoga-poses/upward-plank-pose-hands-chair*

Ustrasana. (2020, December 8). Wild Essence. https://thewildessence.com/ustrasana/

Vincent, J., Copeland, L., & Washburn, L. (n.d.). You-fit exercises for everybody. In *University of Arkansas System.* https://www.uaex.uada.edu/publications/pdf/FSFCS71.pdf

What is chair yoga & what are its benefits. (n.d.). YMCA Whittier. https://ymcawhittier.org/what-is-chair-yoga-benefits/

Will. (2023, April 10). *Top 10 Yoga Poses for Improved Mobility: Unlock Your Body's Potential.* MyYogaTeacher. https://www.myyogateacher.com/articles/yoga-for-improved-mobility

Yoga for arthritis: 9 poses for joint pain relief. (n.d.). Brett Larkin Yoga. https://www.brettlarkin.com/yoga-for-arthritis/

Z Living Staff. (2018, June 8). *Palm Tree Pose | A Powerful Stretch to Detox and Stimulate Digestion.* Z Living. https://www.zliving.com/fitness/yoga/yoga-poses/palm-tree-pose-talasana-97491/

Printed in Great Britain
by Amazon

29039140R00098